D1529842

ANXIETY DISORDERS
IN CHILDREN
AND ADOLESCENTS

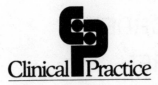

Clinical Practice

Number 22
Judith H. Gold, M.D., F.R.C.P.(C)
Series Editor

ANXIETY DISORDERS
IN CHILDREN
AND ADOLESCENTS

Syed Arshad Husain, M.D., F.R.C.P.(C), F.R.C.Psych.

Professor and Chief
Division of Child and Adolescent Psychiatry
University of Missouri—Columbia
School of Medicine
Columbia, Missouri

Javad H. Kashani, M.D.

Professor of Psychiatry (Child Psychiatry)
Director of Training
Division of Child and Adolescent Psychiatry
University of Missouri—Columbia
School of Medicine
Columbia, Missouri

Washington, DC
London, England

Copyright © 1992 American Psychiatric Press, Inc.
ALL RIGHTS RESERVED
Manufactured in the United States of America on acid-free paper
First Edition
95 94 93 92 4 3 2 1

American Psychiatric Press, Inc.
1400 K Street, N.W., Washington, DC 20005

Library of Congress Cataloging-in-Publication Data

Husain, Syed Arshad.
    Anxiety disorders in children and adolescents / Syed Arshad
      Husain, Javad H. Kashani. — 1st ed.
        p. cm. — (Clinical practice ; no. 22)
      Includes bibliographical references and index.
      ISBN 0-88048-467-5 (alk. paper)
      1. Anxiety in children. 2. Anxiety in adolescence. I. Kashani,
    Javad H., 1937– . II. Title. III. Series.
      [DNLM: 1. Anxiety Disorders—in adolescence. 2. Anxiety Disorders—in infancy & childhood. W1 CL767J no. 22 / WM 172
H969a]
    RJ506.A58H87   1992
    618.92'85223—dc20
    DNLM/DLC
    for Library of Congress   91-22233
                                        CIP

British Library Cataloguing in Publication Data

A CIP record is available from the British Library.

*T*his book is dedicated to our children, Keary and Darius and Fred and Donna, and to their mothers, Jennifer and Soraya, who have been a source of sustained aspiration and guidance.

Contents

Introduction
to the Clinical Practice Series

Over the years of its existence the series of monographs entitled *Clinical Insights* gradually became focused on providing current, factual, and theoretical material of interest to the clinician working outside of a hospital setting. To reflect this orientation, the name of the Series has been changed to *Clinical Practice.*

The Clinical Practice Series will provide readers with books that give the mental health clinician a practical clinical approach to a variety of psychiatric problems. These books will provide up-to-date literature reviews and emphasize the most recent treatment methods. Thus, the publications in the Series will interest clinicians working both in psychiatry and in the other mental health professions.

Each year a number of books will be published dealing with all aspects of clinical practice. In addition, from time to time when appropriate, the publications may be revised and updated. Thus, the Series will provide quick access to relevant and important areas of psychiatric practice. Some books in the Series will be authored by a person considered to be an expert in that particular area; others will be edited by such an expert who will also draw together other knowledgeable authors to produce a comprehensive overview of that topic.

Some of the books in the Clinical Practice Series will have their foundation in presentations at an annual meeting of the American Psychiatric Association. All will contain the most recently available information on the subjects discussed. Theoretical and scientific data will be applied to clinical situations, and case illustrations will be utilized in order to make the material even more relevant for the practitioner. Thus, the Clinical Practice Series should provide educational reading in a compact format especially written for the mental health clinician–psychiatrist.

Judith H. Gold, M.D., F.R.C.P.(C)
Series Editor
Clinical Practice Series

Clinical Practice Series Titles

Treating Chronically Mentally Ill Women (#1)
Edited by Leona L. Bachrach, Ph.D., and Carol C. Nadelson, M.D.

Divorce as a Developmental Process (#2)
Edited by Judith H. Gold, M.D., F.R.C.P.(C)

Family Violence: Emerging Issues of a National Crisis (#3)
Edited by Leah J. Dickstein, M.D., and Carol C. Nadelson, M.D.

Anxiety and Depressive Disorders in the Medical Patient (#4)
By Leonard R. Derogatis, Ph.D., and Thomas N. Wise, M.D.

Anxiety: New Findings for the Clinician (#5)
Edited by Peter Roy-Byrne, M.D.

The Neuroleptic Malignant Syndrome and Related Conditions (#6)
By Arthur Lazarus, M.D., Stephan C. Mann, M.D., and
Stanley N. Caroff, M.D.

Juvenile Homicide (#7)
Edited by Elissa P. Benedek, M.D., and Dewey G. Cornell, Ph.D.

Measuring Mental Illness: Psychometric Assessment for Clinicians (#8)
Edited by Scott Wetzler, Ph.D.

Family Involvement in Treatment of the Frail Elderly (#9)
Edited by Marion Zucker Goldstein, M.D.

Psychiatric Care of Migrants: A Clinical Guide (#10)
By Joseph Westermeyer, M.D., M.P.H., Ph.D.

Office Treatment of Schizophrenia (#11)
Edited by Mary V. Seeman, M.D., F.R.C.P.(C), and Stanley E. Greben,
M.D., F.R.C.P.(C)

The Psychosocial Impact of Job Loss (#12)
By Nick Kates, M.B.B.S., F.R.C.P.(C), Barrie S. Greiff, M.D., and
Duane Q. Hagen, M.D.

New Perspectives on Narcissism (#13)
Edited by Eric M. Plakun, M.D.

**Clinical Management of Gender Identity Disorders in Children
and Adults (#14)**
Edited by Ray Blanchard, Ph.D., and Betty W. Steiner, M.B., F.R.C.P.(C)

Family Approaches in Treatment of Eating Disorders (#15)
Edited by D. Blake Woodside, M.D., M.Sc., F.R.C.P.(C), and Lorie Shek-ter-Wolfson, M.S.W., C.S.W.

Adolescent Psychotherapy (#16)
Edited by Marcia Slomowitz, M.D.

Benzodiazepines in Clinical Practice: Risks and Benefits (#17)
Edited by Peter R. Roy-Byrne, M.D., and Deborah S. Cowley, M.D.

Current Treatments of Obsessive-Compulsive Disorder (#18)
Edited by Michele Tortora Pato, M.D., and Joseph Zohar, M.D.

Children and AIDS (#19)
Edited by Margaret L. Stuber, M.D.

Special Problems in Managing Eating Disorders (#20)
Edited by Joel Yager, M.D., Harry E. Gwirtsman, M.D., and Carole K. Edelstein, M.D.

Suicide and Clinical Practice (#21)
Edited by Douglas Jacobs, M.D.

Anxiety Disorders in Children and Adolescents (#22)
By Syed Arshad Husain, M.D., F.R.C.P.(C), F.R.C.Psych., and Javad Kashani, M.D.

Psychopharmacological Treatment Complications in the Elderly (#23)
Edited by Charles A. Shamoian, M.D., Ph.D.

Chapter 1

Historical Perspectives

*T*he symptoms that we now associate with anxiety disorders were identified over a century ago by DaCosta when he first described the condition "irritable heart" (DaCosta 1871). During World War I, the symptoms of palpitation, dyspnea, and fatigue that characterized this syndrome were accorded such labels as "neurocirculatory asthenia" (Oppenheimer et al. 1918) and "effort syndrome" (Lewis 1919), a term made popular by the belief that the symptoms were precipitated by exercise. A common treatment for this condition was graded exercise, which was done in an effort to increase the patient's tolerance to physical exertion.

As for the existence of anxiety disorder in children, clinicians in the United States were influenced by the views of Benjamin Rush (considered by some to be the father of psychiatry in the United States), who believed that madness in children was rare before puberty because their brains were not yet fully developed (Rubinstein 1948). In Europe, Emminghaus published the first full volume of *Psychic Disturbances of Children* in 1887 and outlined "Psychoneurotic Disorders" of childhood. He described the syndrome of anxiety as "neurasthenia cerebralis" and included under it such symptoms as excessive mental strain, withdrawal, oversensitivity, tearful apprehension, and psychosomatic symptoms. He also ascribed the etiology of the syndrome to neural exhaustion, parental severity, and parental projection of overambitiousness to the child (Harm 1967). Downe in 1887 was probably the first to establish a link between parental anxiety disorder and psychopathology in children (Walk 1964). Theodore Heller established a school in Vienna for children with mental deficiencies and "neurotic" complaints. On the basis of his experiences in that facility he published *Nervous Conditions of Childhood* in 1904, which underscored the prominence of anxious mood in these children.

Freud was the first to propose that the development of cardiorespiratory symptoms could be related to anxiety. His theories of anxiety changed markedly over 40 years. One of his earliest discussions on the manifestations of anxiety concerned hysterical attacks; he viewed "strangulated affect" as a major feature of these attacks (Breuer and Freud 1893). During this same period Freud also discussed neurasthenia, a condition he characterized as an exhaustion of the nervous system in which symptoms of anxiety were prominent (Freud 1895). Freud distinguished neurasthenia from the chronic state of anxiety neurosis, features of which include hypochondria, phobias, anxious expectation, fear of heights, obsessive brooding, and periodic depression.

Freud hypothesized that anxiety-related symptoms could arise psychologically from the inability of the nervous system to respond appropriately to a real or perceived danger. In this case, the individual's response to danger resulted in the accumulation of excitation, which, if overwhelming, may be discharged in the form of anxiety (Freud 1895). Freud believed that anxiety was in fact the discharge of repressed affect: thoughts that were repressed into the subconscious because their content was unacceptable to the individual, only to be later transformed and manifested as anxiety.

Freud maintained that anxiety could develop in the absence of any assumed psychological mechanisms. He postulated that sexual or libidinal energy, if prevented from full expression or discharge, could be transformed directly into anxiety without undergoing psychological transformation. Furthermore, he believed that the anxiety neurosis has no psychical mechanism, and that its specific cause, the accumulation of sexual tension, is produced by abstinence or by unconsummated sexual excitation (Freud 1895). Nemiah (1984) recently pointed out that this biological concept of anxiety is in accordance with the modern concept of the development of panic attacks in the apparent absence of psychological conflict.

Freud (1916–1917) described three types of neurotic anxiety. These correspond to conditions that today would be referred to as phobic disorders and anxiety states, including panic attacks. He described the various manifestations of neurotic anxiety as 1) that which is characterized by a general apprehensiveness or "free-floating" anxiety, referring to this state as "anxious expectation"; 2) that which is attached to particular objects or situations composing the various phobias; and 3) that which is apparently unrelated to any threat of danger and makes its appearance as an "unrelated attack of anxiety." Klein

(1983) notes that Freud recognized the causal relationship between the primary panic attack and the secondary fear of helplessness that leads to the development of avoidant behaviors.

In 1920 Freud presented his theory on traumatic neurosis, stating that the source of the trauma is an excess of stimuli experienced by an individual (Freud 1920). He considered the anxiety dreams of traumatic neurosis to be a retrospective attempt by the organism to master the previously overwhelming stimuli.

Freud also postulated a genetic basis for anxiety (Kedward and Cooper 1966). According to this theory, the state of anxiety is inherited by the individual as a "primeval traumatic experience" handed down from generation to generation. The characteristic form in which anxiety is expressed is determined by the trauma of the birth experience. Later in life, as the mother becomes associated with satisfaction of the infant's basic needs, the untimely absence of the mother during a state of "growing tension due to need" leads to the development of anxiety based on the infant's fear of object loss. The mother's absence then in effect invokes a signal of anxiety; hence, the infant may develop anxiety even in the absence of actual trauma. This signal anxiety can then serve to warn the infant of impending helplessness; adaptive behavior may thus develop to prevent the dangerous situation from recurring.

Freud's theories of anxiety and psychopathology were largely derived from the psychoanalysis of adults, during which childhood experiences were reconstructed. However, at the beginning of this century Freud described the case of little Hans, a 5-year-old suffering from horse phobia (Freud 1909). This case is the first in which Freud applied the psychoanalytic technique of treatment to a child, initiating a technique that required direct observation of the infants and the children in their family and their institution.

A number of child psychoanalysts (Freud 1963; Klein et al. 1952; Mahler et al. 1975) further elaborated the psychoanalytic views of anxiety, both conceptually and clinically. Mahler et al. (1975) postulated a state of symbiosis between mother and infant occurring at about 3 to 18 months of age that allowed the mother to function as an auxiliary ego for the infant and helped the infant to develop ego boundaries. Additionally, Mahler et al. theorized that rejection by or loss of a mother or mothering figure early in life produces panic and anxiety. Anna Freud, another child analyst, identified the developmental sequence by which different forms of anxiety characterize different stages in the development of object relations (Freud 1963). She emphasized the relationship between anxiety and instincts and pointed out that in the early developmental period the intensity of an infant's rage and destructive impulses may leave him or her with a feeling of overwhelming anxiety. Alternatively, Melanie Klein and coworkers (1952) emphasized the struggle between life and death instincts already operating at the time of birth, giving rise to persecutory anxiety.

In summary, Freud's major reformulation of the theory of anxiety (Freud 1926) stimulated considerable research on anxiety, but it did not bring about either consensus or clarity (Yorker and Wiseberg 1976).

Paralleling development of the psychoanalytic theory of anxiety was the research into childhood emotional development and the identification and consolidation of the concepts of "stranger" and "separation" anxieties (Bowlby 1973; Darwin 1872; Ekman et al. 1972; Izard 1971; Watson and Morgan 1917). It is recognized that some seven to nine categories of emotions, including anxiety and distress, are revealed in facial expressions even in blind children (Eibl-Eibesfeldts 1973; Thompson 1941). Both naturalistic and experimental studies have shown that after approximately 6 months of age infants begin to manifest anxiety-like symptoms when their mother leaves them alone, particularly in a strange environment. The development of both stranger and separation anxieties requires the cognitive ability to differentiate facial features, attachment to a caregiver, and normal maturation of the child (Emde et al. 1976).

Alongside the development of psychoanalytic theories of anxiety was the work of behaviorists and the development of theories of learning and conditioning. In 1921 Pavlov induced an "anxiety neurosis" in a dog by presenting it with increasingly difficult and finally impossible problems in stimulus discrimination (Pavlov 1927). Subsequent experiments indicated that dogs with different "personalities" responded differently to the same experimental conditions and stressed genetic mediation of these differences. In the United States Watson and Rayner (1920) produced a phobia of a white rat in an 11-month-old child by conditioning techniques. This phobia subsequently became generalized to a dog, a fur coat, and, to a lesser extent, a Santa Claus beard. Jones (1924) used the technique of systematic desensitization to treat a 3-year-old boy who had a fear of white furry creatures.

Other data that gave impetus to our understanding of anxiety and anxiety disorders resulted from research on anxiety in nonhuman primates. Earlier researchers viewed anxiety as solely a human emotion (Kubie 1953), a view that has now changed after the recent observation that a closely comparable analogue of anxiety (and anxiety disorders) exists in higher primates such as macaque or rhesus monkeys (Suomi 1986). (Anxiety studies in nonhuman primates will be discussed in detail in Chapter 2.)

Along with our rapidly improving understanding of psychopathology in humans, there had been a glaring need for a more adequate and objective classification system for emotional and mental disorders. A number of nosological systems have developed since Kraepelin (1883); throughout the past century anxiety and anxiety disorders have been given a prominent place in all psychiatric classification systems (Anthony 1975).

The first concerted effort to classify anxiety disorders in children was made by the Group for the Advancement of Psychiatry (1966), which termed psychoneurotic disorders as either "psychoneurotic disorder anxiety type" or "psychoneurotic disorder phobic type."

DSM-I (American Psychiatric Association 1952) made no mention of anxiety disorder in children. In DSM-II (American Psychiatric Association 1968) only one condition, "overanxious reaction of childhood or adolescence," was described under behavior disorders. DSM-III and DSM-III-R (American Psychiatric Association 1980, 1987) described three conditions under a broader category of anxiety disorders of childhood and adolescent. These include 1) anxiety disorder, 2) avoidant anxiety disorder, and 3) overanxious disorder. Anxiety is the predominant feature in all three conditions. In the first two conditions situation-specific anxiety is present, whereas the last is associated with generalized anxiety that is not situation-specific.

References

American Psychiatric Association: Diagnostic and Statistical Manual: Mental Disorders. Washington, DC, American Psychiatric Association, 1952
American Psychiatric Association: Diagnostic and Statistical Manual of Mental Disorders, 2nd Edition. Washington, DC, American Psychiatric Association, 1968

American Psychiatric Association: Diagnostic and Statistical Manual of Mental Disorders, 3rd Edition. Washington, DC, American Psychiatric Association, 1980

American Psychiatric Association: Diagnostic and Statistical Manual of Mental Disorders, 3rd Edition, Revised. Washington, DC, American Psychiatric Association, 1987

Anthony JE: Neurotic disorders, in Comprehensive Textbook of Psychiatry. Edited by Freedman AM, Kaplan HI, Sadock BJ. Baltimore, MD, Williams & Wilkins, 1975, p 2143

Bowlby J (ed): Separation Anxiety and Anger (Attachment and Loss Series, Vol 2). New York, Basic Books, 1973

Breuer J, Freud S: On the psychical mechanism of hysterical phenomenon: preliminary communication (1893), in The Standard Edition of the Complete Psychological Works of Sigmund Freud, Vol 2. Translated and edited by Strachey J. London, Hogarth Press, 1955, pp 1–17

DaCosta J: On irritable heart: a clinical study of a functional cardiac disorder and its consequences. Am J Med Sci 61:17–52, 1871

Darwin C: The Expression of Emotions in Man and Animals. London, John Murray, 1872

Eibl-Eibesfeldts J: The expressive behaviors of the deaf and blind-born, in Social Communication and Movement. Edited by Voss Cranach M, Vines I. New York, Academic Press, 1973

Ekman P, Friesan WV, Ellswork PC: Emotion in the Human Face. Guideline for Research and Integration of Findings. New York, Pergamon, 1972

Emde RN, Gaensbauer TJ, Harmon RJ: Emotional Expression in Infancy. New York, International Universities Press, 1976

Freud A: The concept of developmental lines. Psychoanal Study Child 18:245–265, 1963

Freud S: On the grounds for detaching a particular syndrome from neurasthenia under the description "anxiety neurosis" (1895), in The Standard Edition of the Complete Psychological Works of Sigmund Freud, Vol 3. Translated and edited by Strachey J. London, Hogarth Press, 1962, pp 85–117

Freud S: Analysis of a phobia in a five-year-old boy (1909), in The Standard Edition of the Complete Psychological Works of Sigmund Freud, Vol 10. Translated and edited by Strachey J. London, Hogarth Press, 1955, pp 5–147

Freud S: Introductory lectures on psychoanalysis (Part III) (1916–1917), in The Standard Edition of the Complete Psychological Works of Sigmund Freud, Vol 16. Translated and edited by Strachey J. London, Hogarth Press, 1963

Freud S: Beyond the pleasure principle (1920), in The Standard Edition of the Complete Psychological Works of Sigmund Freud, Vol 18. Translated and edited by Strachey J. London, Hogarth Press, 1955, pp 7–64

Freud S: Inhibition, symptoms and anxiety (1926), in The Standard Edition of the Complete Psychological Works of Sigmund Freud, Vol 20. Translated and edited by Strachey J. London, Hogarth Press, 1959, pp 87–175

Group for the Advancement of Psychiatry: Psychopathological Disorders in Childhood: Theoretical Considerations and a Proposed Classification (GAP Report 62). New York, Group for the Advancement of Psychiatry, 1966

Harm E: Origins of Modern Psychiatry. Springfield, IL, Charles C Thomas, 1967

Izard CE: The Face of Emotion. New York, Plenum, 1971

Jones M: A laboratory study of fears. Pedagogical Seminars 31:308–315, 1924

Kedward HB, Cooper B: Neurotic disorders in urban practices: a 3 year follow-up. J Coll Gen Pract 12:148–163, 1966

Klein D: Panic and anxiety (letter). Arch Gen Psychiatry 40:1149, 1983

Klein M, Heimann P, Isaac S, et al: Developments in Psychoanalysis. London, Hogarth Press, 1952

Kraepelin E: Compendium der Psychiatrie. Liepzig, Abel, 1883

Kubie LS: The concept of normality and neurosis, in Psychoanalysis and Social Work. Edited by Heiman M. New York, International Universities Press, 1953

Lewis T: The Soldier's Heart and the Effort Syndrome. London, Shaw, 1919

Mahler MS, Pine F, Bergman A: Psychological Birth of the Human Infant. Symbiosis and Individuation. New York, Basic Books, 1975

Nemiah J: The psychodynamic view of anxiety, in Diagnosis and Treatment of Anxiety Disorder. Edited by Pasnau R. Washington, DC, American Psychiatric Press, 1984, pp 117–137

Oppenheimer BS, Levine SA, Morison R, et al: Report on neurocirculatory asthenia and its management. Military Surgery 42:409–426, 1918

Pavlov IP: Conditioned Reflexes and Psychiatry. New York, Dover, 1927

Rubinstein EA: Childhood mental disease in America: a review of the literature before 1900. Am J Orthopsychiatry 185:314–320, 1948

Suomi SJ: Anxiety-like disorders in young nonhuman primates, in Anxiety Disorders of Childhood. Edited by Gittelman R. New York, Guilford, 1986, pp 1–23

Thompson J: Development of facial expression in blind and seeing children. Arch Psychol (Frankf) 164:1–47, 1941

Walk A: The prehistory of child psychiatry. Br J Psychiatry 110:754–767, 1964

Watson JB, Morgan JJB: Emotional reactions and psychological experimentation. Am J Psychol 28:163–174, 1917

Watson J, Rayner R: Conditioned emotional reactions. J Exp Psychol 3:1–22, 1920

Yorker C, Wiseberg S: A developmental view of anxiety: some clinical and theoretical considerations. Psychoanal Study Child 31:107–135, 1976

Chapter 2

Animal Models of Anxiety

*T*he current explosion of research on the etiological, physiological, and clinical indicators of anxiety disorders has paved the way for the development of an animal model. This trend is further facilitated by an ever-growing fund of knowledge on the cognitive, emotional, social, and physiological development of nonhuman primates (Suomi 1986).

An animal model is defined as an experimental reproduction in nonhumans of the essential features of one of the various human disorders or conditionings (Suomi 1986). The animal model derives its great utility and value from the fact that research animals are not subject to the same limitations as are human subjects. Additionally, the animals' growth rates and shorter life spans facilitate the observation and evaluation of the natural history of a disorder or the long-term effects of a treatment in a short period of time. Conversely, animal models are limited in that most of them are simulative and can be only partially generalized to humans. A few animal models are substitutive, in that cross-species generalization from animals to humans can be made completely. For example, the visual system of chimpanzees is identical to that of humans.

Anxiety and Primates

Anxiety was once viewed as exclusive to humans, who were considered to be the only creatures with sufficient cognitive and emotional ability to experience the anxiety state (Kubie 1953). Research during the past two decades has drastically altered this view. It is now agreed that certain individuals in all advanced primate species (e.g., macaque and rhesus monkeys) manifest behavioral and psychophysiological reactions analogous to anxiety and anxiety disorder in humans.

Definition of Anxiety

Anxiety is an emotional state, a construct encompassing physiological, cognitive, and behavioral components that can be measured. Similar measures are used to observe and assess anxiety in humans and nonhuman primates.

Most studies of anxious behavior in captive rhesus monkeys and other nonhuman primates utilize the same definition of anxiety that is used for humans: "fearful" behavior in the apparent absence of any obvious fear stimulus (Bowlby 1969; Zuckerman and Spielberger 1976).

Separation Anxiety in Young Primates

When separated from their biological mothers, rhesus monkey infants demonstrate a set of behaviors that are similar to those seen in human infants. These behaviors range from facial grimaces, increased contact-seeking and contact-maintaining behaviors, and increased nonnutritive nipple contact. They also show a reduction or disappearance of behaviors such as social play and exploration and locomotion away from the mother.

When separated from their mothers involuntarily, the young primates behave in a manner consistent with a severe fright reaction. They increase their cooing and vocalization and act panicky. This reaction is short-lived and diminishes in intensity when the young primates are returned to the familiar group and surroundings. However, in the ensuing days, weeks, and sometimes even months, they demonstrate a much higher basal level of anxiety-like symptoms. They appear jumpy and on edge, as if suffering from an anxiety attack (Suomi 1981).

Factors Influencing Anxiety Reactions

A number of factors have been identified that influence the intensity and duration of anxiety-like behaviors in young primates. The youngsters who have experienced separation from the mother early in life or who have been separated frequently show more intense anxious behavior. The offspring of neglectful or abusive mothers also have severe responses to separation. The young primates in a social group with unstable dominance hierarchy or where the composition of the group changes frequently also react more adversely than do the ones belonging to a stable environment and hierarchical system.

Age is also an important factor that influences the anxiety-like reaction in nonhuman primates. Juvenile monkeys (1 to 3 years of age) often show regressive behaviors such as clinging to the mother or a peer, and their behavior is markedly agitated. In contrast, regression in the adolescent monkey is limited to milder agitation and stereotypical behavior. Exploration play and sexual or grooming patterns cease in both juvenile and adolescent monkeys (Mineka et al. 1981).

Physiological Correlates

Most animal studies tend to correlate physiological signs with behavior patterns believed to denote anxiety. Increased activity of the adrenocortical system (Coe and Levine 1981; Levine 1983) and elevated heart rate and body temperature (Reite et al. 1981) have been linked with "anxious behaviors." Extreme elevation of plasma cortisone levels, heart rate, and body temperature lasts for a short period after separation. Behavioral recovery precedes adrenocortical system recovery in normal primates. Anxious subjects, however, exhibit consistently higher levels of neurohormonal and sympathetic arousal following challenges.

Individual Differences

Studies have shown that differences exist among individual monkeys in their pattern of response to unusual and strange circumstances. Based on the nature and intensity of their behaviors in the face of adversity, some young monkeys may be differentiated into a timid and anxiety-prone group, with others joining a more outgoing, less cautious group. Longitudinal studies have demonstrated that these differences in physiological and behavioral responses to challenge observed in infancy remain stable across major periods of development (Higley et al. 1984). Monkey infants with highly reactive behavioral responses to stress also tend to have marked physiological responses compared with the responses of their less reactive peers. It is important to note that individual differences in the behavioral expression of anxiety do not begin to stabilize until the second month of life in rhesus monkeys

(Suomi 1983, 1984). Developmentally, this age is roughly comparable to 4 to 8 months of age in human infants.

Monkeys that are not overanxious show a greater initial reaction when involuntarily separated from their caregivers. This reaction takes the form of intense cooing or vocalization. However, plasma cortisone levels remain unchanged (Levine et al. 1984; Suomi 1983). This excessive initial response in the form of cooing is considered to be a species-normative "coping reaction" rather than an index of emotional distress, thus explaining this negative correlation.

In contrast, overanxious young monkeys do not display such reactions. These individual differences have been found to depend on both environmental and genetic factors (Scanlan et al. 1982; Suomi 1981).

Conclusion

The literature reviewed in this chapter indicates that nonhuman primates demonstrate physiological and behavioral reactions that are analogous to anxiety and anxiety disorders in humans. Individual differences exist in these reactions from infancy, the differences remain stable over time, and they are influenced by environmental and genetic factors.

Suomi identifies two general principles relevant to humans that emerge from these studies. First, display of fear and anxiety in certain situations is normal and developmentally appropriate and is most likely shaped by natural selection. A reaction that is appropriate in one situation or at a given stage of development may be quite abnormal in a different context or if displayed by an older individual. Second, there is no reason to believe that highly reactive infants will inevitably develop childhood anxiety disorders (Suomi 1986).

References

Bowlby J: Attachment (Attachment and Loss Series, Vol 1). New York, Basic Books, 1969

Coe CL, Levine S: Normal responses to mother-infant separation in nonhuman primates, in Anxiety: New Research and Changing Concept. Edited by Klein D, Rabkin J. New York, Raven, 1981

Higley JD, Suomi SJ, Delizio RD: Continuity of social separation behaviors from infancy to adolescence. Paper presented at the 7th meeting of the American Society of Primatologists, Acra, CA, 1984

Kubie SL: The concept of normality and neurosis, in Psychoanalysis and Social Work. Edited by Heiman M. New York, International Universities Press, 1953

Levine SA: A psychobiological approach to the ontogeny of coping, in Stress Coping and Development in Children. Edited by Garmezy M, Rutter M. New York, McGraw-Hill, 1983

Levine S, Franklin D, Gonzalez CA: Influence of social variables on the biobehavioral response to separation in rhesus monkey infants. Child Dev 55:1386–1393, 1984

Mineka S, Suomi SJ, Delizio RD: Multiple separations in adolescent monkeys: an opponent-process interpretation. J Exp Psychol [Gen] 110:56–85, 1981

Reite M, Short R, Seiler C, et al: Attachment, loss and depression. J Child Psychol Psychiatry 22:141–169, 1981

Scanlan JM, Suomi SJ, Higley JD, et al: Stress and heredity in adrenocortical response in rhesus monkeys (*Macaca mulatta*). Society for Neuroscience Abstracts 8:461, 1982

Suomi SJ: Genetic, maternal and environmental influences on social development in rhesus monkeys, in Primate Behavior and Psychobiology. Edited by Chiarelli B, Corruccini R. Berlin, Springer-Verlag, 1981

Suomi SJ: Social development in rhesus monkeys: consideration of individual differences, in The Behavior of Human Infants. Edited by Oliverio A, Zapella M. New York, Plenum, 1983

Suomi SJ: The development of affect in rhesus monkeys, in The Psychobiology of Affective Development. Edited by Fox N, Davidson R. Hillsdale, NJ, Lawrence Erlbaum, 1984

Suomi SJ: Anxiety-like disorders in young nonhuman primates, in Anxiety Disorders of Childhood. Edited by Gittelman R. New York, Guilford, 1986

Zuckerman M, Spielberger CD (eds): Emotions and Anxiety. Hillsdale, NJ, Lawrence Erlbaum, 1976

Chapter 3

Epidemiology

*P*sychiatric epidemiology can be defined as the study of the determinants of the incidence and prevalence of mental disorders. Whereas the basis of clinical research is the observation of individual patients, epidemiology requires observation within the communities among which disease occurs. Historically, epidemiology arose from the study of epidemic disease such as plague, cholera, and scurvy, but its scope has now expanded to include all diseases, including psychiatric disorders (Alderson 1976). The implications of this relatively simple definition of epidemiology are widespread. Although it suggests that epidemiology may be used to identify the cause of a given disorder, other intervening factors play an important part. These factors include frequency variations over different periods of time, the characteristics of affected individuals, and the geographical distribution of the disease. A basic premise of epidemiological research is that the distribution of a specific disorder is not randomly determined, but that it varies among subgroups defined by demographic variables such as age, sex, socioeconomic status, etc. Ultimately, knowledge derived from epidemiological studies may aid in the planning of services for the prevention, control, and treatment of disease.

A limited number of epidemiological studies exist for psychiatric diagnoses, and fewer still specifically address anxiety disorders. A review of child psychiatric epidemiological research (Schwartz-Gould et al. 1981) showed that most studies reported global estimates of maladjustment rather than estimates of specific disorders. Orvaschel and Weissman (1986) reviewed seven studies that estimated the prevalence of childhood anxiety. They noted the difficulties encountered in attempting to obtain a composite picture of the epidemiology of anxiety in children; informants varied across studies, and different instruments, as well as different methods of assessment, were used. This review also indicated that few data were available on specific anxiety disorders in children and adolescents and that existing data were limited to estimates of symptom prevalence.

In this chapter, we will review the literature on the prevalence of anxiety disorders (both general and specific) in 1) the general population and 2) the clinical sample. Specific demographic determinants of mental disorders such as age, sex, race, and socioeconomic status will be included in this review.

Community Samples

The classic epidemiological study by Lapouse and Monk (1958) examined the frequency of a wide range of child behaviors and characteristics. The sample consisted of children between the ages of 6 and 12 years, from 482 randomly selected households. Lapouse and Monk reported that the children in their study had a 43% prevalence rate of "many fears and worries." Black children had more fears and worries (63%) than white children (44%), children in low socioeconomic groups had more fears and worries (50%) than children in higher socioeconomic groups (36%), and 50% of the girls had seven or more fears and worries compared with only 36% of the boys. The prevalence rates decreased as the child aged, and the symptoms were not correlated with other indicators of psychopathology.

Agras et al. (1969) conducted a two-stage epidemiological study of fears and phobias in a random sample of 325 adults and children. Information was obtained by an interview that listed 40 common fears and investigated their presence, intensity, and so forth. (A separate questionnaire including 21 items was used for children under the age of 14 years.) A psychiatrist then identified those respondents believed to be phobic based on the questionnaire results. Overall, the prevalence rate for all phobias was 7.7%. In 74.7% of the cases the phobia was reported to be mildly disabling, and in 0.2% of the cases the phobia was reported to be severely disabling.

Werry and Quay (1971) used a sample of 1,753 children in kindergarten through second grade to obtain prevalence data. The overall prevalence for anxiety/fearfulness was reported to be 16% for boys and 17% for girls. They also found that anxiety symptoms showed a steady decline from 5 through 7 years of age.

Richman et al. (1975) used a random sample of 705 3-year-olds in a study of the prevalence of behavior problems. These researchers identified 2.5% of the boys and 2.6% of the girls as worriers. The prevalence of fears in the sample was 8.0% for boys and 17.2% for girls.

Earls (1980) used another sample of 100 3-year-old children in his study of the prevalence of behavior problems. His findings revealed that 7% of the children had moderate to severe behavior problems. He reported the prevalence of several worries to be 7.5% for boys and 8.6% for girls and the prevalence of several fears to be 25.5% for girls but only 3.7% for boys.

Kastrup (1976) did a cross-sectional survey of 175 preschool children aged 5 to 6 years. He reported the prevalence of nightmares to be 11% for boys and 5% for girls, the prevalence of fears to be 3% for boys and 5% for girls, and the prevalence of fear of separation to be 12% for boys and 16% for girls.

Abe and Masui (1981) investigated sex differences in the prevalence of fears and anxiety symptoms in a sample of 2,500 individuals aged 11–23 years. The researchers did not find persistent sex differences in anxiety symptoms. All of the fears were found to be more prevalent in girls, with the exception of fear of talking, which was more frequently reported by boys. Specific prevalence estimates were not reported by these researchers.

All of these general population findings were based on studies that preceded the DSM-III (American Psychiatric Association 1980). In a more recent study by Anderson and colleagues (1987), DSM-III disorders in 792 11-year-old children from the general New Zealand population were studied. DSM-III diagnoses were based on information obtained from structured child interviews and standardized parent and teacher questionnaires. The 1-year prevalence rates for anxiety disorders were 3.5% (separation anxiety disorder), 2.9% (overanxious disorder), 2.4% (simple phobia), and 0.9% (social phobia). All of the anxiety disorders had an overrepresentation of females, with the exception of overanxious disorder.

Kashani and Orvaschel (1988) reported the 6-month period prevalence of anxiety disorders in a community sample of 150 adolescents aged 14 to 16 years. Diagnoses were based on structured psychiatric interviews, a psychiatrist's review of the data, and DSM-III criteria. Findings showed that 8.7% of the adolescents met criteria for one or more anxiety diagnoses and were identified as "cases" (based on need for treatment). When the need for treatment and impairment of functioning were not considered, the prevalence doubled; 17% of all adolescents were diagnosed as having some type of anxiety disorder.

More specific anxiety disorders were investigated in a community-based developmental study of children and adolescents in three age groups (8-, 12-, and 17-year-olds) (Kashani et al. 1989). Anxiety was found to be the most frequently reported type of psychopathology in all three age groups. Content area scores and item frequencies indicated that anxiety symptoms such as separation concerns decreased with age. This is in contrast to specific fears and social embarrassment, both of which increased with age. This finding suggests that while rates of anxiety remain the same, the focus changes with increasing age, from family-oriented to interpersonal/peer concerns. While both males and females showed similar trends over time with respect to most types of anxiety, only females become more anxious over time about competence.

A two-stage epidemiological survey of the prevalence of mental disorders in children in a Puerto Rico community was carried out by Bird and his colleagues (1988). The ages of the children ranged from 4 to 16 years. The Child Behavior Checklist (CBCL) was used as a screening instrument during the first stage, and children were evaluated clinically during the second stage. (Because the operational definitions and the systems for measurement of child psychopathology are still ill-defined, the researchers in this study used a combination of measures to operationally define mental disorder). Compliance rates were 92.2% ($n = 777$) for the first stage and 87.7% ($n = 386$) for the second stage. The second-stage sample consisted of all the positive screens from the CBCL results in the first stage, as well as 20% of the negative screens. Clinical assessments for the second-stage sample included the administration of the Diagnostic Interview Schedule for Children (DISC-C) and parents (DISC-P). The psychiatrists also scored each child on the Children's Global Assessment Scale (CGAS). Subjects who met DSM-III criteria for one or more disorders and who had a CGAS score of less than 61 were considered to be "definitely" maladjusted (cases); those subjects who met DSM-III criteria for disorder and who had a CGAS score between 61 and 70 were considered as "possibly" maladjusted (not definite cases); and those subjects whose CGAS score was over 70 were considered as noncases.

The 6-month weighted prevalence rates of the most common diagnostic categories for both cases and possible cases were estimated.

Anxiety disorders were classified into two types: separation anxiety disorder and simple phobias. (The milder forms of these disorders were less likely to warrant clinical attention and thus were excluded from this study.) A diagnosis of separation anxiety disorder was made in 4.7% (weighted percentage) of cases, while 2.6% of the cases had a diagnosis of simple phobia. In contrast, 2.1% of the possible cases had a diagnosis of separation anxiety disorder and 1.3% of the possible cases had a diagnosis of simple phobia.

The demographic correlates of these diagnoses in this child population were consistent with other findings in the epidemiological literature; psychopathology was more strongly associated with males and lower socioeconomic status. Some disorders such as separation anxiety disorder peaked in the 6-year-old to 11-year-old age group. The authors suggest that the prevalence of maladjustment in the Puerto Rican children is generally consistent with prevalence rates obtained in other community surveys.

Flament et al. (1985) investigated obsessive-compulsive disorder by surveying more than 5,000 students in a New Jersey school district. Their findings established a minimal prevalence rate of 0.33% for obsessive-compulsive disorder in the general population.

The study by Whitaker et al. (1990) focused on psychiatric disorders. Recent data from the Epidemiological Catchment Area Study suggest that young adults with an earlier anxiety or depressive disorder are at increased risk for substance abuse.

The sample in the present study consisted of all the students enrolled in the 9th through 12th grades (5,596 students) in a single New Jersey county in October 1984. The DSM-III diagnosis of generalized anxiety disorder was assigned in one of two ways: 1) by the field clinician at the time of the interview and 2) by computer scanning of the precoded interview responses for the core of necessary symptoms for the disorder.

Weighted prevalence rates for generalized anxiety disorders revealed that 4.6% of the females had the diagnosis and 1.8% of the males had the diagnosis. Hence, girls were significantly more likely to meet criteria for generalized anxiety disorder (odds ratio = 3.6, $P < .05$). The sexes were equally at risk for panic disorder (0.7% for females and 0.4% for males) and obsessive-compulsive disorder (1.8% for females and 0.6% for males).

Only two of the subjects diagnosed with generalized anxiety disorder were hospitalized. However, many came to the attention of professionals.

In the Ontario Child Health Study (Offord et al. 1987), 6-month prevalence rates were compiled for individual disorders (conduct disorder, hyperactivity, emotional disorder, and somatization) and for one or more disorders by sex and age.

Focusing on emotional disorders, it was found that both age and sex significantly affected the prevalence rates. In the 4-year-old to 11-year-old age group, the rates for boys and girls were almost identical (10.2% for boys and 10.7% for girls). The rate dropped to 4.9% for boys and increased to 13.6% for girls in the 12-year-old to 16-year-old age group. Overall, emotional disorder was 2.8 times more prevalent among older Ontario girls than among older boys. For specific disorders, the authors determined the prevalence of overanxious disorder and separation anxiety disorder to be 3.6% and 2.4%, respectively, among young people aged 12–16 years (Bowen et al. 1990).

Suicidal behavior in normal schoolchildren was the focus of a study by Pfeffer et al. (1984). A total of 101 children aged 6–12 years were selected by stratified random sampling from a roster of pupils in a large urban community. There were 71 boys and 30 girls (mean age = 9.7 years) chosen for the investigation, and the racial/ethnic distribution was 75.2% white and 24.8% black. The DSM-III diagnoses for the school children were compared with those of 65 inpatients. By applying DSM-III criteria to the clinical data, both the therapist on the inpatient unit and the interviewer of the schoolchildren determined the diagnoses. Overanxious disorder, the most frequent Axis I diagnosis, was present in 27.7% ($n = 28$) of the schoolchildren. In contrast, only 9.2% ($n = 6$) of the inpatients had a diagnosis of overanxious disorder. One explanation offered by the authors for this difference between the two populations is that, in the inpatient sample, other symptoms may completely dominate the child's presentation and bias the clinician in arriving at a diagnosis. This study furthers our knowledge of the prevalence of overanxious disorder within both the general and the clinical population. However, the use of a structured standard psychiatric interview would have improved the reliability of the epidemiological data collected.

Clinical Population

Epidemiological data must be derived from both treated and untreated population samples in order to obtain unbiased estimates of the prevalence of psychiatric disorders. Hence, in contrast to the studies previously described, the following investigations report prevalence data on anxiety disorders from inpatient samples.

Last et al. (1987a) evaluated the DSM-III diagnostic categories of separation anxiety disorder and overanxious disorder in a clinical sample of 91 children and adolescents. A total of 69 children (76%) met DSM-III criteria for separation anxiety disorder ($n = 22$), overanxious disorder ($n = 26$), or both ($n = 21$). Further examination of children with separation anxiety disorder (47%) indicated that the majority were under the age of 13 years (91%) and were Caucasian (86%). Sex distribution of the disorder was roughly equivalent for boys and girls. Also, 75% of the children diagnosed as having separation anxiety disorder came from families of low socioeconomic status. According to this study, overanxious disorder was as common as separation anxiety disorder, with 52% ($n = 47$) of the patient sample meeting DSM-III criteria for the disorder. However, children with overanxious disorder were more likely than children with separation anxiety disorder to have an additional concurrent anxiety disorder, usually simple phobia or panic disorder. In contrast to children with separation anxiety disorder, children with overanxious disorder differed on several demographic variables: children with overanxious disorder were usually over the age of 13 years (69%), and 80% came from families of middle to high socioeconomic status. Hence, because of the differing characteristics of the two anxiety disorders, results from this study support the DSM-III distinction between overanxious disorder and separation anxiety disorder.

Overanxious disorder was also studied in a sample of 57 outpatient boys aged 8 to 12 years (Mattison and Bagnato 1987). Sixteen of the 57 boys were diagnosed as having overanxious disorder, with the mean age of this group being 10.2 years. The boys were primarily Caucasian, and their average Hollingshead socioeconomic level was IV. The purpose of this study was threefold: 1) to determine any validating relationship between overanxious disorder and profile types on the parental CBCL; 2) to distinguish boys with overanxious disorder from boys with dysthymic disorder or attention-deficit hyperactivity disorder (ADHD) based on cutoff techniques for the Child Behavior Profiles (CBP) and the Revised Children's Manifest Anxiety Scale (RCMAS); and 3) to investigate the potential of combining cutoff procedures for the CBP and RCMAS to improve the classification of overanxious disorder in children.

Convergent and discriminant validity were demonstrated. The overanxious group showed the greatest number of high correlations with the CBP schizoid or anxious type. However, none of this group had a CBP type that was most highly correlated with either the hyperactive or delinquent type. A clinically derived DSM-III diagnosis of overanxious disorder in boys aged 8–12 years was also found to be empirically verified by a pathologically elevated score on the worry/oversensitivity factor of the RCMAS. The conclusions of this study underscore the importance of multimethod, empirical assessment in substantiating overanxious disorder.

Measurement of anxiety was investigated in a study by Hoehn-Saric et al. (1987). The sample consisted of 63 children (average age 11.6 years, with a range of 7–17 years) selected from a total of approximately 200 admissions to a child and adolescent psychiatric inpatient unit over a 10-month period. All children were assessed using 1) the Children's Anxiety Evaluation Form (CAEF), 2) the self-rated State-Trait Inventory for Children (STAIC), and 3) the RCMAS. The CAEF, based on history, signs, and symptoms obtained through semistructured interviews, was developed in order to obtain clinically meaningful assessments of anxiety, which are often lacking when self-rating instruments are used.

Within the total sample, there were sufficient numbers of patients in five diagnostic groups to allow statistical comparison among the three anxiety measures. Results showed that CAEF scores differentiated patients diagnosed as having anxiety disorders from those who were diagnosed as having oppositional disorder, conduct disorders (aggressive and nonaggressive), and dysthymic disorders. The STAIC and RCMAS failed to differentiate diagnostic groups (despite a positive correlation between CAEF scores on one hand, and STAIC trait scores and RCMAS on the other). The anxiety measures were assessed for differences between the 41 boys and 22 girls. Only on the CAEF were significant differences between gender found ($P < .0001$), with boys having an average score of 6.80 (maximum = 12) and girls having an average score of 3.73. In summary, this study showed the utility of the CAEF by demonstrating the CAEF's ability to differentiate anxiety disorders from other diagnostic categories. Hence, the importance of a semistructured interview as opposed to a self-rating scale is supported.

Children with separation anxiety ($n = 48$) and a group of children with school phobia ($n = 19$) were compared on various characteristics such as demographic data, symptoms, concurrent psychiatric disorders, and maternal psychiatric illness in a study by Last et al. (1987b). Findings revealed that, in general, children with separation anxiety disorder were female, prepubertal, and from lower socioeconomic status families, while school phobic children tended to be male, postpubertal, and from higher socioeconomic status families. Furthermore, 92% of the children with separation anxiety disorder ($n = 44$) met criteria for at least one concurrent disorder, compared to 63% ($n = 12$) of the school phobic group. Finally, mothers of children with separation anxiety disorder had a rate of affective disorder four times greater than that of mothers of children with school phobia. In summary, the results showed that the two anxiety disorders differed on a number of variables, thus supporting the use of DSM-III criteria for differentially diagnosing separation anxiety disorder and school phobia.

Costello et al. (1988) utilized a psychiatric interview specifically designed for epidemiological studies to estimate the prevalence of specific DSM-III disorders in a large sample of United States children. A two-stage design was used in which all children aged 7 to 11 years visiting a primary care clinic formed the sample to be screened using the CBCL. A subgroup consisting of severely disturbed children was selected for detailed psychiatric interviews and follow-up. Using sampling fractions of the children scoring above and below the screening cutoff point of the CBCL, prevalence rates for the entire sample of 789 children were estimated. (These prevalence estimates were calculated for the total screened sample of 789 children by weighing the proportion of screen-positive and screen-negative children in the interviewed sample of 300 children by the appropriate sampling fraction.) The DISC-C and DISC-P were used to provide the data needed for making DSM-III diagnoses. Prevalence rates were reported on the basis of three systems of data aggregation: "parent diagnoses" (DISC-P), "child diagnoses" (DISC-C), and "parent or child diagnoses" (either DISC-P or DISC-C).

Anxiety disorders investigated included separation anxiety, avoidant disorder, overanxious disorder, simple phobia, social phobia, agoraphobia, and panic disorder. Prevalence rates derived from parents' responses to the DISC-P ranged from 0.4% to 3.0%. Prevalence rates obtained from the children's responses to the DISC-C ranged from 4.1% to 6.7%. Prevalence rates obtained from the parent or the child ranged from 1.0% to 9.2%. After combining the emotional and behavioral diagnoses into five groups (conduct disorder, ADHD, oppositional disorder, anxiety disorder, and affective disorders), weighted prevalence estimates for the screened sample indicated that both parents and children reported anxiety disorders more frequently (5.3% and 8.9%, respectively) than any others, both alone and in conjunction with other disorders.

Risk factors associated with parent reports of DSM-III emotional disorders (as opposed to behavioral disorders) included a high level of stress in the girls' lives, but this was not true for the boys. (Since parents reported few depressive disorders in their children, this association with stress primarily relates to the anxiety disorders.) Based on children's reports of DSM-III emotional disorders, data showed that girls with family difficulties were also more likely to report emotional problems. Boys' risk of emotional problems was increased by high stress levels in the lives of the parents or the children and also by having a mother with a high level of concurrent psychiatric distress. Repeating a grade increased the risk of a self-reported emotional disorder threefold for both sexes. Also, emotional disorders were twice as likely in younger children (7 to 9 years old) than in the 10- to 11-year-old age group. This difference is primarily caused by a higher rate of separation anxiety in the younger children. A final factor that increased the likelihood of both parental and child reports of emotional and behavioral disorders was a recent stressful event in the child's life. This large-scale study increases our knowledge of the prevalence of risk factors for anxiety disorders and other psychiatric disorders in a primary care population.

The largest systematic study of children and adolescents with obsessive-compulsive disorder was carried out at the Child Psychiatry Branch of the National Institute of Mental Health (Leonard and Rapoport 1989). The sample was composed of 70 children with obsessive-compulsive disorder. The mean age of onset was 10.2 years, with males having an earlier age of onset than females (9.8 years vs. 11.0 years, respectively). Males outnumbered females by more than 2:1.

Finally, a study by Kashani et al. (1989) systematically identified the severity of anxiety in a sample of 100 inpatient children (ages 7–12 years) by means of multiple informants. Those children who were diagnosed as having an anxiety disorder (overanxious, separation anxiety, or phobia) as revealed by the parent's report (Diagnostic Interview for Children and Adolescents, Parents' Version) and the children's report (Diagnostic Interview for Children and Adolescents) were considered to have the most serious type of anxiety ($n = 21$, 21%). Children reported to have an anxiety diagnosis by only one informant (parent or child) ($n = 48$, 48%) were considered to have "possible" anxiety. Finally, a third group, without any of the three anxiety disorders according to either informant ($n = 31$, 31%), completed the sample.

The responses obtained from multiple informants were validated by means of a variety of well-standardized anxiety scales: anxious and nonanxious children had significantly different total scores on the RCMAS. That is, the severity of the anxiety was reflected in the high scores on the RCMAS for the anxious group only. Also, the Piers-Harris Anxiety factor and the Personality Inventory for Children (PIC) anxiety scale provided further validation for a clear distinction between the anxious and nonanxious children.

Additional findings indicated that the parents of children with severe anxiety had more anxiety, obsessive-compulsive symptoms, or depressive symptoms (as revealed by the Symptom Checklist–90) than did the parents of children with no anxiety diagnosis. Finally, as severity of anxiety within the sample increased, so also did the prevalence of dysthymia and negative life events. In conclusion, this study further elucidated the nature of anxiety through the use of dual informants who categorized subjects into groups based on the severity of their anxiety.

Conclusions

On the basis of a literature review across community and clinical samples, it appears that anxiety disorders of all types are quite prevalent, ranging from 0.9% of a community sample (social phobia) to 52% of a clinical sample (separation anxiety disorder). It is important to note, however, that discrepancies in prevalence rates from our two types of population samples may be due not only to the type of sample used but also to the different diagnostic criteria and methodologies employed. Still another problem with the present information regarding anxiety disorders is that many researchers report only specific anxiety disorder prevalence rates, as opposed to overall and combined prevalence rates (e.g., Anderson et al. 1987). Because there is invariably an overlap among anxiety disorders, we are not able to obtain consistent and accurate data on the overall prevalence of anxiety disorders for the purpose of comparisons among studies.

On the whole, girls tend to report more fears and worries than do boys (e.g., Earls 1980; Lapouse and Monk 1958), although there are a few exceptions to this finding (e.g., Kastrup 1976; Last et al. 1987a). In addition, prevalence reports regarding gender vary according to the type of anxiety disorder and demographic variables (e.g., age and socioeconomic status of the child's family).

Anxiety, specifically separation anxiety, generally declines in prevalence with age (e.g., Kashani et al. 1989), although there is some indication that specific fears or phobias become more dominant as the child ages (e.g., Last et al. 1987a). Children with overanxious disorder have also been found to be older than children with other anxiety disorders (e.g., Last et al. 1987a).

Finally, when racial and socioeconomic status data are reported, it seems that there are many discrepancies among prevalence data. Again, demographic reports depended on the type of anxiety disorder investigated and the sample used. For example, in the community sample of Lapouse and Monk (1958), black children had more fears and worries than did white children, and low socioeconomic status children had more fears and worries than did high socioeconomic status children. Last et al. (1987a) found that children diagnosed as having separation anxiety were primarily Caucasian and frequently came from families of low socioeconomic status. In contrast, those children with overanxious disorder came from families of middle to high socioeconomic status. Hence, the relationship of these demographic variables to anxiety disorders is still unclear.

Due to the DSM-III changes in anxiety diagnostic criteria, several researchers have published data in support of the validity of anxiety disorders. For example, Last et al. (1987a) supported the DSM-III distinction between separation anxiety disorder and overanxious anxiety disorder by showing that the two disorders differed with respect to several demographic variables. Likewise, Mattison and Bagnato (1987) studied empirical assessment of overanxious disorder in boys.

Future research should include the use of multiple informants in diagnosing anxiety disorder to avoid inaccurate reporting of prevalence rates. Through the use of multiple informants, the most serious cases can be identified so that the severity of the anxiety can be quantitated for investigational purposes. Finally, overall prevalence rates and the overlap among anxiety disorders should be added to the epidemiological reports of specific anxiety disorder prevalence rates.

References

Abe K, Masui T: Age-sex trends of phobic and anxiety symptoms. Br J Psychiatry 138:297–302, 1981

Agras S, Sylvester D, Oliveau D: The epidemiology of common fears and phobias. Compr Psychiatry 10:151–156, 1969

Alderson M: Introduction to Epidemiology. London, Macmillan, 1976, p 1

American Psychiatric Association: Diagnostic and Statistical Manual of Mental Disorders, 3rd Edition. Washington, DC, American Psychiatric Association, 1980

Anderson JC, Williams S, McGee R, et al: DSM-III disorders in preadolescent children. Arch Gen Psychiatry 44:69–76, 1987

Bird HR, Canino G, Rubio-Stipec M, et al: Estimates of the prevalence of childhood maladjustment in a community survey in Puerto Rico. Arch Gen Psychiatry 45:1120–1126, 1988

Bowen RD, Offord DR, Boyle MH: The prevalence of overanxious disorder and separation anxiety disorder: results from Ontario Child Health Study. J Am Acad Child Adolesc Psychiatry 29(5):753–758, 1990

Costello EJ, Costello AJ, Edelbrock C, et al: Psychiatric disorders in pediatric primary care. Arch Gen Psychiatry 45:1107–1116, 1988

Earls F: The prevalence of behavior problems in three year old children: a cross-cultural replication. Arch Gen Psychiatry 37:1153–1157, 1980

Flament M, Rapoport J, Berg C, et al: A controlled trial of clomipramine in childhood obsessive-compulsive disorder. Psychopharmacol Bull 21:150–152, 1985

Hoehn-Saric E, Maisami M, Wiegard D: Measurement of anxiety in children and adolescents using semistructured interviews. J Am Acad Child Adolesc Psychiatry 26(4):541–545, 1987

Kashani JH, Orvaschel H: Anxiety disorders in mid-adolescence: a community sample. Am J Psychiatry 145:960–964, 1988

Kashani JH, Orvaschel H, Rosenberg TK, et al: Psychopathology among a community sample of children and adolescents: a developmental perspective. J Am Acad Child Adolesc Psychiatry 28:701–706, 1989

Kastrup M: Psychic disorders among pre-school children in a geographically delimited area of Aarhus county, Denmark. Acta Psychiatr Scand 54:29–42, 1976

Lapouse R, Monk MA: An epidemiologic study of behavior characteristics in children. Am J Public Health 48:1134–1144, 1958

Last CG, Hersen M, Kazdin AE, et al: Comparison of DSM-III separation anxiety and overanxious disorders: demographic characteristics and patterns of co-morbidity. J Am Acad Child Adolesc Psychiatry 26(4):527–531, 1987a

Last CG, Francis G, Hersen M, et al: Separation anxiety and school phobia: a comparison using DSM-III criteria. Am J Psychiatry 144:653–657, 1987b

Leonard HL, Rapoport JL: Anxiety disorders in children and adolescents, in American Psychiatric Press Review of Psychiatry, Vol 8. Edited by Tasman A, Hales RE, Frances AJ. Washington, DC, American Psychiatric Press, 1989, pp 162–179

Mattison RE, Bagnato SJ: Empirical measurement of overanxious disorder in boys 8 to 12 years old. J Am Acad Child Adolesc Psychiatry 26(4):536–540, 1987

Offord DR, Boyle M, Szatmari P, et al: Ontario Child Health Study, II: six-month prevalence of disorder and rates of service utilization. Arch Gen Psychiatry 44:832–836, 1987

Orvaschel H, Weissman MM: The epidemiology of anxiety disorders in children, in Anxiety Disorders of Childhood. Edited by Gittelman R. New York, Guilford, 1986, pp 58–72

Pfeffer CR, Zuckerman S, Plutchik R, et al: Suicidal behavior in normal school children: a comparison with child psychiatric inpatients. J Am Acad Child Psychiatry 23(4):416–423, 1984

Richman N, Stevenson JE, Graham PJ: Prevalence of behavior problems in three-year old children: an epidemiologic study in a London borough. J Child Psychol Psychiatry 16:277–287, 1975

Schwartz-Gould M, Wunsch-Hitzig R, Dohrenwend B: Estimating the prevalence of childhood psychopathology: a critical review. J Am Acad Child Psychiatry 20:462–476, 1981

Werry JS, Quay HC: The prevalence of behavior symptoms in younger elementary school children. Am J Orthopsychiatry 41:136–143, 1971

Whitaker A, Johnson J, Shaffer D, et al: Uncommon trouble in young people: prevalence estimates of selected psychiatric disorders in a non-referred adolescent population, Arch Gen Psychiatry 47:487–496, 1990

Chapter 4

Diagnosis and Assessment of Anxiety Disorders in Children and Adolescents

Anxiety is defined as "apprehension, tension, or uneasiness that stems from the anticipation of danger, which may be internal or external" (American Psychiatric Association 1980, p. 354). Anxiety may be focused on an object, situation, or activity that is avoided (phobia), or it may be unfocused (free-floating anxiety).

Anxiety is present in all emotional disorders, and it is integral to all theories of psychopathology (Gittelman 1986). Dimensionally, therefore, anxiety figures in the differential diagnosis of all disorders of childhood, adolescence, and adulthood. Among the illnesses grouped conceptually as "anxiety disorders," the distinctiveness of anxiety lies in the fact that it is the predominant clinical feature.

Anxiety is expressed as a fear or dread of a future event that a person perceives as dangerous, overwhelming, or unmanageable. Whereas fear is considered a normal reaction to an objectively dangerous situation, anxiety may occur either as unrelated to external stress or as an exaggerated response to ordinary or mild stress. The conceptual distinction between anxiety and fear relates to their unique precipitating factors. Functionally, however, the manifestations of both fear and anxiety are so similar that beginning with DSM-III the distinction between the two has been de-emphasized. The apprehension that characterizes both fear and anxiety emanates from anticipated danger without regard for whether the threat is internal or external.

Anxiety as Symptom or Disorder

It is important to define a number of concepts that are frequently used when describing anxiety. Anxiety as a symptom may be seen in other clinical entities (such as obsessive-compulsive disorder) as an emotion, a psychophysiological response, or an indescribable behavior (Werry 1986). As a symptom, anxiety may present itself as an isolated emotion or as part of a broader group of symptoms comprising a disorder. In turn, a disorder is a medical concept with a universally consistent clinical picture, epidemiology, etiology, natural history, and response to treatment.

Anxiety as Trait or State

Distinction should also be made between anxiety as a trait and anxiety as a state. Anxiety as a trait is a rather stable intrinsic feature of one's personality and can neither be precipitated by an internal event nor, in most instances, be ameliorated by a therapeutic intervention. In contrast, a state of anxiety occurs in reaction to an external identifiable event, is of variable intensity, and is transient (Gittelman-Klein 1988). Although the clinical manifestations of anxiety—whether as a symptom, trait, state, or disorder—may be similar and can be consistently measured, these four concepts are not interrelated and do not shift from one to another during the clinical course of an illness. For example, a chronic anxiety disorder may initially present as a trait. However, a more detailed evaluation often reveals that the symptoms of the anxiety disorder are specific to an experience or object (e.g., social phobias) and are not pervasive and generalized as in the case of trait anxiety.

Assessment

Werry (1986) identifies four objectives in assessing anxiety that are dependent on the theoretical frame of reference and the purpose of the assessor. These include diagnosis, treatment plan formulation, evaluation of treatment, and research. The diagnostic purpose of assessment is to establish a clinical judgment concerning the presence or absence of anxiety based on currently accepted criteria. Formulation of a treatment program follows from diagnosis, and evaluation of such treatment requires measurements of anxiety in order to assess the efficacy of the treatment. Further assessment of anxiety for research purposes exceeds these diagnostic and treatment objectives and requires greater consensus among researchers as to the methodology and quality of the measures used.

Werry (1986) has also discussed the characteristics of a good measure and has identified four desirable features. These include "explication," "comprehensiveness," "practicality and ethical acceptability," and "reliability and validity." A measuring tool should be clear in its use and interpretation so that the interassessor variability is reduced to a minimum. It should encompass all aspects of anxiety, including developmental stages as they apply to symptoms, disorder traits, state, or behavior. An assessment tool should be easily available, rapid, inexpensive, and nonintrusive so as to be practical and acceptable to all concerned. The precision, reliability, or internal consistency of a method of measurement pertains to the degree to which it gives the same answers regardless of frequency of usage by either the same or different people. Validity, on the other hand, refers to how well a tool measures what it is intended to measure. Methods of measurement that are not reliable consequently cannot be valid, although the converse is not true.

Personality Tests as Measure of Anxiety

Advances in statistical methodology, such as factor analysis, have facilitated the development of a number of personality measures that often include an anxiety scale. Disadvantages of the early tests, such as the California Test of Personality (Thorpe et al. 1953a), included their inordinate length and lack of comprehensive assessment; they also required rather advanced reading skills on the part of the child being evaluated (Klein 1988). Personality tests also pose another disadvantage. Since they are self-report measures and since each child applies a different standard to evaluate his or her own anxiety pertaining to a situation or object, personality tests are often subject to a rater's bias. Personality tests, therefore, have only limited utility in the assessment of anxiety in children (Klein 1988). However, it is worth mentioning a few personality tests for children that are currently in vogue.

California Test of Personality

This is one of the oldest and most widely used personality tests in the United States. The California Test of Personality has four forms. Its primary form was developed for children in kindergarten through third grade (Thorpe et al. 1953a); the elementary form, for fourth to sixth graders (Thorpe et al. 1953b); the intermediate form, for seventh to tenth graders (Clark et al. 1953); and the secondary form, for ninth graders through college students (Tiegs et al. 1953). The specific scale addressing issues related to anxiety is called "freedom from nervous symptoms" and explores somatic complaints such as headaches, stomachaches, colds, etc.

Cattell's Personality Questionnaire

Cattell and his colleagues at the University of Illinois have been applying factor analysis to facilitate the definition and measurement of anxiety. They have devised three self-rating personality questionnaires, one for each different age group. They include the Early School Personality Questionnaire (Cattell and Coan 1979) for children aged 6–8 years, the Children's Personality Questionnaire (Porter and Cattell 1979) for children aged 8–12 years, and the High School Personality Questionnaire (Cattell and Cattell 1979) for adolescents. Several personality traits appear to relate to the anxiety experiences and thus measure some aspects of anxiety. The questionnaires have been criticized for their lack of ability to address specific areas of function (Thorndike 1978).

Eysenck Personality Questionnaire

The child version of the Eysenck Personality Questionnaire (Eysenck and Eysenck 1975) has a neuroticism scale; however, it is not designed to evaluate information about fears, anxiety, and worries. The measure also lacks norms, and the validity of this instrument for measuring anxiety is questionable.

Interviews

The personal interview is one of the oldest and most widely used devices to measure personality and psychopathology. In spite of the interview's largely subjective nature, a well-trained interviewer can function as a reasonably good measuring instrument. Interviewers have the advantage of flexibility in exploring a wide range of feelings related to personal experiences, situations, and relationships. The interview also allows the interviewers not only to hear what the person is saying but also to observe bodily, facial, and vocal reactions and also more intangible behaviors. The interviews are usually used by the clinicians to round out a clinical picture of psychopathology.

The interview as an assessment tool has many limitations. It requires some judgment rating or interpretation by the interviewer; hence, the skills and the experience of the interviewer become important variables. It is also difficult to express the results of an interview in quantitative terms, rendering data comparison impossible. When combined with other objective tests, however, interviews can provide more valid judgments than either type alone.

Typically, an interview to assess anxiety and anxiety disorders involves both the child or adolescent and his or her parents. Parental interview focuses on obtaining the chief complaint, history of present illness, and ameliorating and exacerbating factors. A detailed developmental history including dates of various milestones, information about attachment, and the quality of bonding should always be obtained from the parents. A history of major life events should be documented. The quality of the mother-child relationship should be explored, and the reaction of the child when first separated from the mother should be obtained. The first major separation usually occurs when the child starts a day-care program or enters preschool. The parents of anxious children and children with separation anxiety often report severe reactions to such separation. Information about primary temperament, fears, phobias, worries, and nightmares should also be obtained.

Family history of psychiatric illness, particularly of anxiety disorder in close relatives, should also be documented.

In the individual interview of the child, an attempt should be made to explore fears, fantasies, worries, and phobias that the child is encountering. The child should be closely observed during separation from his or her parents, as well as throughout the interview itself.

Structured Interviews

There have been numerous efforts to systematize this interview technique into a reliable and standardized tool to screen large populations for psychiatric disorders. The earliest of the structured interviews was developed by Rutter and his colleagues (Graham and Rutter 1968; Rutter and Graham 1968) for use in the Isle of Wight studies. This interview yields a single overall category of anxiety, among other psychiatric disorders in children.

Since DSM-III, a number of structured interviews have been developed. Each of these has a number of questions devoted to the screening of anxiety disorders. Three of these structured interviews will be discussed briefly in this chapter.

Diagnostic Interview for Children and Adolescents (DICA). This structured interview was developed by Herjanic and her colleagues at Washington University (Herjanic and Campbell 1977; Herjanic and Reich 1982; Reich et al. 1982). The 1981 version of the DICA is modeled after the Diagnostic Interview Schedule (DIS; Robins et al. 1981). The DICA is a highly structured interview designed for research purposes and can be used by clinicians. Since it does not require any clinical judgment on the part of the interviewer, it can also be administered by trained lay interviewers. The DICA can be used for children aged 6 to 17 years. A version (DICA-P) is also administered to parents to further evaluate the child.

The DICA and DICA-P have three components. The first component is common to both versions and is administered conjointly to the child and the parent. This part consists of 19 questions, focusing on an introduction to the structured interview process and obtaining general demographic information. The child's version (part two) consists of 247 questions. Completion of this portion requires about 60 to 90 minutes. However, since the questions are grouped according to specific disorders, selected or abridged portions of the interview can also be administered. For example, questions 158–173 are devoted to separation anxiety disorder. Part two of the DICA-P is no different from part two of the DICA with respect to content, but it is written in the third person so that the same questions can be asked of the parents about the child.

Part three of the DICA includes observational items, while part three of the DICA-P focuses on birth, early development, and medical and family histories.

Data on test-retest reliability and parent-child agreement are available for the DICA and are claimed to be high (Herjanic and Reich 1982). The DICA is considered to be a well-written and scientifically sound instrument; as an added advantage, it can be administered by a lay interviewer. However, it is considered to be a less sensitive indicator of change during follow-up because of its dichotomous positive/negative scoring system and its lack of symptom severity rating (Kashani and Orvaschel 1988).

Diagnostic Interview Schedule for Children (DISC). The Diagnostic Interview Schedule for Children is modeled after the Diagnostic Interview Schedule for Adults (Robins et al. 1981). The current version of the DISC was developed by Costello et al. (1984) while under contract to the National Institute of Mental Health. Like the DICA, the DISC is also highly structured and designed for large-scale epidemiological surveys and can be administered by trained lay interviewers. It is suitable for use in children aged 6 to 17 years and also has a parent version (DISC-P). The DISC has 264 items, and the DISC-P has 302 items. Each version takes 60 to 70 minutes to complete.

The items on the DISC and DISC-P are precoded and the questions are rated as "not true" (0), "somewhat true" (1), "very" or "often true" (2), or no (0)/yes (2). The severity of symptoms is weighed as 0, 1, or 2. The DISC screens all childhood diagnostic categories listed in DSM-III, including separation anxiety disorder, overanxious disorder, phobic disorder, panic disorder, and obsessive-compulsive disorder. Unlike the DICA, questions are not grouped according to the diagnostic categories, although the specific questions for a particular diagnosis can be lifted from the main text and administered. Algorithms are provided for obtaining computerized diagnoses based on the DISC interview data. Interrater reliability for symptom scores averages 0.98 (Costello et al. 1984). The parent-child agreement is poor for an as-yet unknown reason.

Kiddie-Schedule for Affective Disorder and Schizophrenia (K-SADS). The K-SADS is a modification for children of the Schedule for Affective Disorder and Schizophrenia used in adults (Endicott and Spitzer 1978). It was originally developed by Puig-Antich and Chambers (1978) for the assessment of ongoing episodes of psychiatric disorder in studies of the treatment of childhood depression. The K-SADS is suitable for children aged 6 to 17 years. Administration requires a trained clinician and lasts approximately 60 minutes.

The first portion of the K-SADS is unstructured, during which the history of the present illness is obtained along with a description of the ongoing episodes, particularly those segments deemed most severe.

The second part is very structured and consists of 200 specific symptoms or behaviors identifying a number of DSM-III conditions, including separation anxiety, panic, phobias, generalized anxiety disorder, and obsessive-compulsive disorder. The third and final part consists of 16 observational items and the children's version of the global assessment scale, both of which are completed by the interviewer. The K-SADS has a 6- to 7-point severity rating with specific criteria for rating. There is an epidemiological version of the K-SADS (K-SADS-E). The K-SADS-E was developed in order to assess a disorder over time, including exploration of the past history.

The K-SADS has generated data on test-retest reliability, mother-child agreement, and interrater reliability. Interrater reliability ranged from 0.65 to 0.96, and mother-child agreement ranged from 0.08 to 1.0 (Chambers et al. 1985). Anxiety diagnosis also demonstrated low test-retest reliability (Kashani and Orvaschel 1988).

In summary, development of the semistructured and the structured interviews represents efforts to standardize the interview technique for research purposes. Each interview tool is designed for a specific purpose. These interviews are useful in obtaining reliable and more comprehensive assessment of the signs and symptoms of psychiatric disorders; however, their validity as diagnostic tools is hotly debated (Werry 1986).

Anxiety Scales

Most anxiety scales are self-reports and are designed to explore worries, fears, and phobias.

The earliest effort to develop an anxiety scale for children was made by Castaneda et al. (1956), who adapted the Taylor Manifest Anxiety Scale for Adults for use in children and called it the Children's Manifest Anxiety Scale (CMAS). In developing an anxiety scale for adults, Taylor (1953) selected those 50 questions from the Minnesota Multiphasic Personality Inventory (Hathaway and McKinley 1951) that she and her coworkers considered to be the most discriminating between anxious and nonanxious individuals. This scale will be discussed in detail later in this chapter. More recently, Cattell et al. (1976) developed a 40-item anxiety scale, the Institute of Personality and Ability Testing (IPAT) Anxiety Scale, items of which were selected from a broad-based high school personality questionnaire (Cattell and Cattell 1979).

The State-Trait Anxiety Inventory for Children (Spielberger 1973) is a self-rating scale that requires the child to report how he or she feels both at the specific time of reporting (state) and in general (trait). This scale was designed to assess what the CMAS failed to assess, i.e., the response to acute stress. However, the validity of this scale in differentiating state from trait anxiety has been actively debated (Johnson and Melamed 1979).

Children's Manifest Anxiety Scale—Revised (CMAS-R)

The original CMAS consisted of 42 yes/no items and also had a lie scale to assess the respondents' degree of honesty. The anxiety score is simply summed from the total number of "yes" answers.

A revised version of CMAS is now available that includes 25 items from the original scale and 9 additional questions comprising the new lie scale (Reynolds and Richmond 1984). The CMAS-R is suitable for first- through twelfth-grade students. The first and second graders need oral administration since the language used in the items requires third grade or above word attack and comprehension skills.

Factor analysis studies of CMAS-R (Reynolds and Richmond 1984) have identified three factors: factor 1 correlates with physiological signs of anxiety; factor 2, with worry and oversensitivity; and factor 3, with cognitive anxiety (fear/concentration). These factors are similar to ones generated by the original scale (Finch et al. 1974). This finding indicates that the construct validity for CMAS-R is high. Further evidence in support of this validity was provided by Reynolds (1980), who reported high correlation between CMAS-R and the scores for trait anxiety on the State-Trait Anxiety Inventory for Children (Spielberger 1973). CMAS-R has good test-retest reliability and correlates modestly with other similar scales (Johnson and Melamed 1979; Werry 1978). Werry (1978) also found that while the CMAS-R may discriminate between normal persons and various clinical populations, it remains insensitive to stress. Hence, caution has been suggested in drawing conclusions from CMAS scores (Klein 1988).

Rating Scales and Symptom Checklists

Rating scales are a partial solution to the problem of expressing interview data in objective fashion. Rating scales may be used to record data derived from the interviews or from informal observations. Several types of rating scales are in use. The simplest form lists a number of personality characteristics, such as honesty, reliability, and emotionality, and asks a rater who is familiar with the person to rate each characteristic on a scale (e.g., from 1 to 7). Another type of rating scale provides the rater with a number of alternative descriptions and requires from the rater the most applicable alternative; it is possible to convert the results to numerical scores on either a 5-point or a 7-point scale. These scales are usually factor analyzed, and some also provide an anxiety scale.

The rating scales are criticized for their lack of an anchor, effectively allowing different raters to use inconsistent criteria for presence, frequency, and severity. They are also criticized for their use of inaccurate descriptive terms and interpretations that are considered to be too far removed from the clinical situation. Hence, they have been regarded as not helpful in the development of treatment strategies (Conners and Werry 1979; Mash and Terdal 1981a; Wells 1981).

Louisville Behavior Checklist (LBCL)

One of the oldest rating scales, the LBCL (Miller 1967a, 1967b) has an anxiety factor consisting of 11 items: "headaches," "migraine headaches," "stomachache," "somatic fear of school," "worries," "guilt," "complains not loved easily," "feels pain more," "says picked on," "feels inferior," and "cries." The parents rate each item by checking "yes" or "no." This scale was developed for clinically referred boys aged 6 to 12 years and therefore rates anxiety relative to that observed in other patients rather than to that observed in normal populations. This checklist has also been criticized because the anxiety factor does not contain several important items reflecting anxiety. Because of these deficiencies, the LBCL was revised to improve internal consistency and face validity; this newer version is termed the Fear Scale (Miller et al. 1971). This updated new scale has 18 items that include specific fears and items on general anxiety and separation anxiety.

Child Behavior Checklist

This checklist developed by Achenbach (1978) has limited value for anxiety assessment. An anxiety factor was determined for girls aged 4–5 years and 12–16 years but not for girls aged 6–11 years. For boys the anxiety factor was determined only for 6- to 11-year-olds. These and other inconsistencies minimize the Child Behavior Checklist's utility in the assessment of anxiety in children.

Behavioral Assessment of Anxiety Disorders

Behavioral methods of anxiety assessment differ significantly from previously described approaches in that they focus on the observation and recording of behaviors as they occur. Typically, target behaviors are defined first, followed by their eliciting stimuli and contingencies. Length and location of the observation and identity of the observer are also predetermined; target behaviors are then recorded as they occur.

A number of behavioral methods developed in the past decade represent a significant advancement in the assessment of anxiety. For details the readers are referred to Mash and Terdal (1981a), Wells (1981), O'Leary and Johnson (1979), and Werry (1978). Techniques such as behavioral interviews (Mash and Terdal 1981b), the Behavior Avoidance Test (Barrios et al. 1981), and the Echobehavioral Assessment (Wahler 1980; Wahler et al. 1976) are noteworthy.

The behavioral methods have shown high reliability and utility, as well as high relevance to treatment. Their disadvantage is that they are very difficult to administer, requiring a great deal of time and energy on the part of the clinician. They are thus impractical for use in clinical practice (Barrios et al. 1981; Wells 1981; Werry 1978).

Psychological Tests

Both intelligence (e.g., Wechsler Intelligence Scale for Children, Revised) and projective tests (Rorschach, Apperception Test) have been used in the past to assess anxiety in children. The validity of these tests is questionable, however, since all the studies utilizing these methods were published before the current criteria for anxiety disorders were established (Gittelman-Klein 1988). For a review of the role of cognitive and projective tests in the assessment of anxiety disorders in children, the readers are referred to the work of Gittelman (1980) and O'Leary and Johnson (1979).

Physiological Methods of Assessment of Anxiety

Physiological measures are based on the common observation that anxiety is associated with a number of somatic changes involving various body systems. These systems (and respective changes) were reviewed by Lader (1980) and include cardiovascular (increased pulse rate and blood pressure and acral vasoconstriction), respiratory (increased respiration rate, poor utilization of inspired oxygen), endocrine (elevated serum cortisol, 17-hydroxycorticosteroids and aldosterone, and blood and urine catecholamines), musculoskeletal (increased amplitude of finger tremors, increased muscle tension), and pupillary (longer dilatation duration) changes. Electroencephalographic changes include decreased alpha and increased beta rhythms and diminished contingent negative variation. Palmar sweat glands show increased conductance, increased spontaneous fluctuation in conductance, and slower habituation to novel stimuli.

Individuals with anxiety disorders consistently show higher absolute values for a given parameter in response to an acute stress and a slower return to basal levels before removal of the stress (Lader 1980). In reviewing numerous studies, Lader (1980) concluded that anxious patients exhibit heightened levels of alertness, arousal, and preparedness in all the physiological modalities listed above.

Studies of physiological measures in children are scant. What data exist indicate that children follow adult patterns (Barrios et al. 1981; Wells 1981). However, more research is needed before any firm conclusions can be drawn.

The critics of physiological measures and the resultant arousal concept identify a number of problems with this approach (Barrios et al. 1981), such as unreliability of measures across individuals and across situations. Certainly these measures are more useful for research and hold little promise for the clinicians.

Conclusion

The instruments that are currently available to measure anxiety and to identify anxiety disorders in children have limited value. These instruments should be used by clinicians only as an adjunct to their clinical impression.

References

Achenbach TM: The child behavior profile, 1: boys aged 6–11. J Consult Clin Psychol 46:478–488, 1978

American Psychiatric Association: Diagnostic and Statistical Manual of Mental Disorders, 3rd Edition. Washington, DC, American Psychiatric Association, 1980

Barrios BA, Hartmann DP, Shigetomi C: Fears and anxieties in children, in Behavioral Assessment of Childhood Disorders. Edited by Mash EJ, Terdal LG. New York, Guilford, 1981, pp 259–304

Castaneda A, McCandless B, Palermo D: The children's form of the Manifest Anxiety Scale. Child Dev 27:317–326, 1956

Cattell RB, Cattell MD: The High School Personality Questionnaire. Champaign, IL, The Institute for Personality and Ability Testing, 1979

Cattell RB, Coan RW: The Early School Personality Questionnaire. Champaign, IL, The Institute for Personality and Ability Testing, 1979

Cattell RB, Krug SE, Scheier IH: IPAT Anxiety Scale. Champaign, IL, The Institute for Personality and Ability Testing, 1976

Chambers WJ, Puig-Antich J, Hirsch M, et al: The assessment of affective disorders in children and adolescents by semi-structured interview. Arch Gen Psychiatry 42:696–702, 1985

Clark WW, Tiegs EW, Thorpe LP: California Test of Personality Intermediate Form AA. Monterey, CA, McGraw-Hill, 1953

Conners CK, Werry JS: Pharmacotherapy, in Psychopathological Disorders of Childhood, 2nd Edition. Edited by Quay HC, Werry JS. New York, John Wiley, 1979, pp 336–386

Costello AJ, Edelbrock CS, Duncan MK, et al: Diagnostic Interview Schedule for Children. Washington, DC, National Institute of Mental Health, 1984

Endicott J, Spitzer RL: A diagnostic interview: the SADS. Arch Gen Psychiatry 35:837–853, 1978

Eysenck HJ, Eysenck SBG: Eysenck Personality Questionnaire (Junior). San Diego, CA, Educational and Industrial Testing Service, 1975

Finch AJ, Kendall PC, Montgomery LE: Multidimensionality of anxiety in children: factor structure of the Children's Manifest Anxiety Scale. J Abnorm Child Psychiatry 2:331–336, 1974

Gittelman R: The role of psychological tests for differential diagnosis in child psychiatry. J Am Acad Child Psychiatry 19:413–438, 1980

Gittelman R: Childhood anxiety disorders: correlates and outcomes, in Anxiety Disorders of Childhood. Edited by Gittelman R. New York, Guilford, 1986, pp 101–125

Gittelman-Klein R: Childhood anxiety disorders, in Handbook of Clinical Assessment of Children and Adolescents, Vol II. Edited by Kestenbaum CJ, Williams DT. New York, New York University Press, 1988, pp 722–742

Graham P, Rutter M: The reliability and validity of the psychiatric assessment of the child, II: interview with the parents. Br J Psychiatry 114:581–592, 1968

Hathaway SR, McKinley JC: The Minnesota Multiphasic Personality Inventory Manual, Revised Edition. New York, The Psychological Corporation, 1951

Herjanic B, Campbell W: Differentiating psychiatrically disturbed children on the basis of a structured interview. J Abnorm Child Psychol 5:127–134, 1977

Herjanic B, Reich W: Development of a structured psychiatric interview for children: agreement between child and parent on individual symptoms. J Abnorm Child Psychol 10:307–324, 1982

Johnson SB, Melamed BG: Assessment and treatment of children's fears, in Advances in Clinical Child Psychology, Vol 2. Edited by Lahey BB, Kazdin AE. New York, Plenum, 1979, pp 107–139

Kashani JH, Orvaschel H: Anxiety disorders in mid-adolescence: a community sample. Am J Psychiatry 145:960–964, 1988

Klein RG: Childhood anxiety disorders, in Handbook of Clinical Assessment of Children and Adolescents. Edited by Kestenbaum CJ, Williams DT. New York, New York University Press, 1988, pp 722–742

Lader MH: The psychophysiology of anxiety, in Handbook of Biological Psychiatry, II: Brain Mechanisms and Abnormal Behavior—Psychophysiology. Edited by Van Praag HM, Lader MH, Rafaelsen OJ, et al. New York, Marcel Dekker, 1980

Mash EJ, Terdal LG: Behavioral assessment of childhood disturbance, in Behavioral Assessment of Childhood Disorders. Edited by Mash EJ, Terdal LG. New York, Guilford, 1981a

Mash EJ, Terdal LG (eds): Behavioral Assessment of Childhood Disorders. New York, Guilford, 1981b

Miller LC: Louisville behavior checklist for males, 6–12 years of age. Psychol Rep 21:885–896, 1967a

Miller LC: Dimensions of psychopathology in middle children. Psychol Rep 21:897–903, 1967b

Miller LC, Barrett DL, Hampe E, et al: Revised anxiety scales for the Louisville Behavior Checklist. Psychol Rep 29:503–511, 1971

O'Leary KD, Johnson SB: Psychological assessment, in Psychopathological Disorders of Childhood, 2nd Edition. Edited by Quay HC, Werry JS. New York, John Wiley, 1979, pp 210–246

Porter RB, Cattell RB: The Children's Personality Questionnaire. Champaign, IL, The Institute for Personality and Ability Testing, 1979

Puig-Antich J, Chambers WJ: Schedule for Affective Disorders and Schizophrenia for School-Age Children (Present Episode Version) (K-SADS-P). Unpublished manuscript, 1978

Reich W, Herjanic B, Welner Z, et al: Development of a structured psychiatric interview for children: agreement on diagnosis comparing child and parent interviews. J Abnorm Child Psychol 10:325–336, 1982

Reynolds CR: Concurrent validity of What I Think and Feel: The Revised Children's Manifest Anxiety Scale. J Consult Clin Psychol 48:774–775, 1980

Reynolds CR, Richmond BO: Revised Children's Manifest Anxiety Scale. Los Angeles, CA, Western Psychological Services, 1984

Robins LN, Helzer JE, Croughan J, et al: National Institute of Mental Health Diagnostic Interview Schedule. Arch Gen Psychiatry 38:381–389, 1981

Rutter M, Graham P: The reliability and validity of the psychiatric assessment of the child, I: interview with the child. Br J Psychiatry 114:563–579, 1968

Spielberger CD: Manual for the State Trait Anxiety Inventory for Children. Palo Alto, CA, Consulting Psychologists Press, 1973

Taylor JA: A personality scale of manifest anxiety. J Abnorm Soc Psychol 48:285–290, 1953

Thorndike RL: Critique, in The Eighth Mental Measurements Yearbook. Edited by Buros OK. Lincoln, University of Nebraska, 1978, p 766

Thorpe LP, Clark WW, Tiegs EW: California Test of Personality. Primary Form. Monterey, CA, McGraw-Hill, 1953a

Thorpe LP, Clark WW, Tiegs EW: California Test of Personality. Elementary Form. Monterey, CA, McGraw-Hill, 1953b

Tiegs EW, Clark WW, Thorpe LP: California Test of Personality. Secondary Form. Monterey, CA, McGraw-Hill, 1953

Wahler RG: The insular mother: her problems in parent-child treatment. J Appl Behav Anal 13:207–220, 1980

Wahler RG, House AE, Stambaugh EE: Ecological Assessment of Child Problem Behavior. New York, Pergamon, 1976

Wells KC: Assessment of children in outpatient settings, in Behavioral Assessment: A Practical Handbook, 2nd Edition. Edited by Hersen M, Bellak AS. New York, Pergamon, 1981, pp 484–533

Werry JS: Measures in pediatric psychopharmacology, in Pediatric Psychopharmacology: The Use of Behavior Modifying Drugs in Children. Edited by Werry JS. New York, Brunner/Mazel, 1978, pp 29–78

Werry JS: Diagnosis and assessment, in Anxiety Disorders of Childhood. Edited by Gittelman R. New York, Guilford, 1986, pp 73–100

Chapter 5

Classification of Anxiety Disorders

*C*antwell and Baker (1985) have discussed in detail the advantages of classifying psychiatric disorders in children and adolescents as well as the principles used in various classification systems. Briefly, the most important purposes of classification include the ability to systematize collected clinical data and to communicate such data to clinicians, researchers, and other interested parties in an organized fashion. Other advantages include prediction of future patterns, development of scientific theories, treatment planning, and qualification for specialized services.

There are many acceptable classification systems of psychiatric disorders. The two most common are categorical and dimensional systems. The DSM and International Classification of Diseases (ICD) classifications are the prime examples of the categorical system. Developed after the medical model, the categorical system establishes clinical criteria for a particular diagnostic category, with diagnosis being made only when those criteria are met. In contrast, the dimensional system utilizes statistical methods to define dimensions of behavior, which are then scored to produce a profile. The dimensional system is becoming increasingly popular and owes its popularity to workers such as Achenbach (1982), one of the leading proponents of the multivariate statistical approach. Some workers are now attempting to use multivariate techniques in combination with a categorical approach to achieve a more effective classification system (Pfohl and Andreasen 1978).

Anxiety as a clinical symptom has been found to dominate various childhood psychiatric disorders and has gained prominence in most classifications of mental diseases (Anthony 1975). In this chapter only a few of the more well-known classifications of anxiety disorders will be discussed.

GAP Classification

The Group for the Advancement of Psychiatry (GAP) gathered together a group of well-known experts in child and adolescent psychiatry, established collaboration, worked with other related disciplines for years, and finally in 1966 produced a monograph entitled *Psychopathological Disorders in Childhood* (Group for the Advancement of Psychiatry 1966). This monograph represented the first concerted effort to classify psychiatric disorders in children and adolescents. It proposed the following major categories of psychiatric conditions: healthy responses, reactive disorders, developmental deviations, psychoneurotic disorders, psychotic disorders, brain syndromes, mental retardation, and other disorders. These categories are arbitrarily arranged in a hierarchy ranging from healthy responses through mild to more severe psychological disorders. Conditions in which somatic factors predominate the clinical picture are ranked last. Two disorders (psychoneurotic disorder, anxiety type, and psychoneurotic disorder, phobic type) top the list of anxiety disorders under the broader category of psychoneurotic disorders.

The GAP reserves the term "psychoneurotic disorders" for those in whom an unconscious conflict exists over the handling of sexual and aggressive impulses; this conflict remains active and unresolved, although removed from awareness by the mechanism of repression (Group for the Advancement of Psychiatry 1966, p. 57). In psychoneurotic disorder, anxiety type, the anxiety arising from the unconscious internalized conflict appears to break through into awareness. The anxiety is free floating and is perceived as an intense and diffuse feeling of apprehension or impending disaster. Caution must be exercised in differentiating anxiety neurosis from acute panic state, which is classified under reactive disorders.

In the psychoneurotic disorder, phobic type, the child is said to unconsciously displace his or her original conflict onto an object or a situation in the external environment that has symbolic significance for him or her, resulting in avoidance of these objects or situations.

In the third condition, psychoneurotic disorder, obsessive-compulsive type, the anxiety produced by the unconscious conflicts is neutralized by the occurrence of thoughts (obsessions) of acts or impulses (compulsion) to act, or both, which are isolated from the original unacceptable impulse. Manifest behaviors such as complete obedience and compliance to parental wishes are opposite to the unconscious wishes of defiance and anger. If interfered with, the ritualistic behaviors such as touching, counting, handwashing, and so forth produce severe anxiety.

The GAP classification also identifies a fourth condition, "anxious personality," under the broader category of "personality disorders." Personality disorders are characterized by fixed or chronic pathological traits that have become ingrained in the personality structure. Children with anxious personality disorder are chronically tense and apprehensive over new situations "often related to their extraordinarily vivid fantasies" (p. 69). The anxiety exhibited, however, is not crippling, as it is in a child with anxiety neurosis.

The "overly inhibited personality" also seems to be relevant to the discussion of anxiety disorders under the GAP classification. The children in this category are extremely shy and experience conscious anxiety. They show marked constriction of personality functions such as inhibition of motor function and reduction of speech; the latter may take the form of elective mutism. Unlike children with schizoid personality, these children long for warm and meaningful relationships but are inhibited from achieving them. These children are less inhibited in familiar surroundings, such as the home environment.

ICD System

The ICD system is a more elaborate system of classification, not only of mental diseases but also of medical and other morbid conditions, injuries, and causes of death. It is a statistical system rather than a nomenclature of diseases. The system is organized into 17 major sections, with section V devoted to mental disorders.

The ICD system has been regularly revised. In 1900 the first revision conference of the "International List of Causes of Death" was held in Paris. None of the first four revisions of the ICD system included mental disorders as a separate section. The fifth revision (World Health Organization 1938) had only a single three-digit category called "Diseases of the Nervous System and Sense Organs," under which were four subcategories: "mental deficiency," "schizophrenia," "manic depressive psychosis," and "all other mental disorders." ICD-6 (World Health Organization 1948), for the first time, provided a separate section on mental disorders (Section V).

The international community of psychiatrists considered ICD-6 (World Health Organization 1948) and ICD-7 (World Health Organization 1955) unsatisfactory, and a major revision was urged. This was finally accomplished by a group of experts convened by the World Health Organization in 1965; as a result, ICD-8 (World Health Organization 1967) was published. ICD-8 lists two conditions specific to children and adolescents: mental retardation and behavior disorders of childhood. The ICD-9 (World Health Organization 1975) reflects the expanding nature of the field, the accumulation of new knowledge, and a response by the international community to the growing need for a uniform nomenclature. More conditions specific to childhood and adolescents, such as "disturbance of emotion specific to childhood and adolescence," were also added.

Anxiety Disorders in ICD-9

In ICD-8 anxiety disorders were listed under the broader category "Neurosis, Personality Disorders and Other Non-Psychotic Mental Disorders." In ICD-9 the term "neurosis" is altered to "neurotic disorder" and a number of conditions are included under it. These include anxiety states, hysteria, phobic states, obsessive-compulsive disorders, neurotic depression, neurasthenia, depersonalization syndrome, hypochondriasis, and other neurotic disorders. The common threads in all these conditions are the absence of a demonstrable organic basis for the condition, the presence of impaired insight, and disorganization of personality. Principal manifestations include excessive anxiety, hysterical symptoms, phobias, obsessive-compulsive symptoms, and depression. Four conditions listed above have anxiety as a partial or dominant feature of the clinical picture and will be briefly defined herein.

Anxiety state.   Anxiety is the main clinical feature, is generally diffuse, and is not attributable to any real danger. Anxiety may occur as a persistent state or may recur as acute attacks, escalating to the point of panic.

Phobic state.   In this condition there is an abnormal dread and fear of specific situations or objects in response to a wider range of circumstances.

Obsessive-compulsive disorder. In this disorder intense anxiety appears when an attempt is made to dispel the unwelcome thoughts, urges, and actions that are the hallmark of this condition.

Neurotic depression. In this condition there is a disproportionate depressive response following a distressing experience, and anxiety is frequently present, presenting a mixed clinical picture of anxiety and depression.

There are two other conditions in ICD-9 that include anxiety as part of the clinical picture and are listed under "adjustment reactions." These include "adjustment reaction with predominant disturbance of other emotions" and "adjustment reaction with mixed disturbance of emotion and conduct." Separation anxiety of abnormal magnitude in children is listed in ICD-9 under adjustment reaction with a predominant disturbance of other emotions. Overanxious reaction of childhood or adolescence is included in ICD-9 under "disturbance of emotions specific to childhood and adolescence."

ICD-9 has been used infrequently in the diagnosis of children and adolescents; hence, no published reliability or validity data are currently available. The classification system also lacks operational criteria and is empirical rather than developmental.

Preparations are already well under way to revise ICD-9, and ICD-10 is expected to be published in 1992, around the same time as DSM-IV. A draft of ICD-10 for field trials has been circulated since 1986 (World Health Organization 1987), with a separate subsection for "behavioral and emotional disorders with onset specific to childhood and adolescence." This subsection includes hyperkinetic disorder, conduct disorder, mixed disorder of conduct and emotion, emotional disorder with onset specific to childhood, disorder of social functioning with onset specific to childhood or adolescence, tic disorders, other behavioral and emotional disorders with onset usually occurring during childhood, and unspecified behavioral or emotional disorder with onset in childhood or adolescence.

Childhood Anxiety Disorder in Draft of ICD-10

Childhood anxiety disorders in ICD-10 are listed under "emotional disorders with onset specific to childhood" and include 1) separation anxiety disorder, 2) phobic disorder of childhood, and 3) social sensitivity disorder. The ICD-10 draft offers diagnostic guidelines and a differential diagnosis for each of these conditions.

The Isle of Wight System

This system, developed by Rutter (Rutter 1976; Rutter et al. 1976) for an epidemiological study, has only one category of anxiety disorder. All the dysphorias are lumped into "emotional disturbance." Although this system has by far the greatest validity and reliability, it has been criticized for its simplicity, and its adequacy for the need of child psychiatry has been debated.

The DSM System and Anxiety Disorders in Children

DSM-I (American Psychiatric Association 1952) was a product of the work done by a committee appointed in 1946 by the American Psychiatric Association (APA) and chaired by Dr. Raines. The committee solicited input from the membership by distributing copies of the proposed nomenclature to about 10% of the APA's membership. DSM-I represented a major improvement over the standard classified nomenclature of diseases previously published in 1933; however, it gave no consideration to childhood psychiatric conditions except for mental deficiency.

The first revision of DSM-I, DSM-II, was developed by an APA committee chaired by Dr. Gruenberg. DSM-II (American Psychiatric Association 1968) recognized specific childhood psychiatric disorders under a single category of "behavior disorders of childhood and adolescence," which has seven subcategories. These include hyperkinetic reaction, withdrawal reaction, overanxious reaction, runaway reaction, unsocialized aggressive reaction, group delinquent reaction, and other reaction. The overanxious reaction of childhood and adolescence most closely resembles anxiety disorder in childhood and adolescence. Adult anxiety disorders in DSM-II are included under the category "neurosis" and include anxiety reaction, phobic reaction, and obsessive-compulsive reactions. These diagnoses could also be applied to children and adolescents.

DSM-III

DSM-III (American Psychiatric Association 1980) for the first time contained a separate comprehensive section on the psychiatric conditions of infancy, childhood, and adolescence. DSM-III also assigned a distinct position to anxiety disorder of childhood or adolescence as a freestanding psychiatric condition of childhood. DSM-III divides anxiety disorders into separation anxiety disorder, avoidant disorder, and overanxious disorder. The adult categories of anxiety disorders such as phobic disorder, obsessive-compulsive disorder, generalized anxiety disorder, and typical anxiety disorder can also be used in children. Certain adjustment disorders under DSM-III classification also include anxiety in the clinical picture.

The DSM-III classification of childhood anxiety disorders has been criticized because of the lack of scientific data validating these classification schemes (Gittelman 1986). Since the publication of DSM-III in 1980, however, a number of trials have been conducted in an effort to assess the reliability of this classification of the childhood anxiety disorders. A large-scale test-retest reliability study of these disorders conducted by Last et al. (1987b) showed excellent rates of agreement for separation anxiety disorder (kappa = .81) and overanxious disorder (kappa = .82) and moderately high agreement for avoidant disorder (kappa = .64).

Last and her colleagues (1987a, 1987c, 1987d) have also conducted validity studies of separation anxiety disorder and overanxious disorder. They found that the two disorders differ significantly across several dimensions including age, social class, and presence of a coexisting anxiety disorder. Significant differences were also found between separation anxiety disorder and school phobia disorder in regard to sex distribution, pubertal status, and socioeconomic background. The children with separation anxiety disorder differed from the children with phobic disorder in their symptomatology, comorbidity, and history of maternal psychiatric illness. Differences in the patterns of comorbidity are also found between children with a primary diagnosis of separation anxiety disorder and those with a primary diagnosis of overanxious disorder (Last et al. 1989). These authors also found statistically significant differences in the types of fears endorsed by children with separation anxiety and those endorsed by children with overanxious disorder.

According to Last and Francis (1988), these findings provide preliminary support for the validity of separation anxiety disorder and overanxious disorder as two distinct diagnostic entities.

DSM-III-R (American Psychiatric Association 1987) has retained all the categories of anxiety disorders presented in DSM-III.

References

Achenbach TM: Developmental Psychopathology, 2nd Edition. New York, John Wiley, 1982, pp 547–576

American Psychiatric Association: Diagnostic and Statistical Manual: Mental Disorders. Washington, DC, American Psychiatric Association, 1952

American Psychiatric Association: Diagnostic and Statistical Manual of Mental Disorders, 2nd Edition. Washington, DC, American Psychiatric Association, 1968

American Psychiatric Association: Diagnostic and Statistical Manual of Mental Disorders, 3rd Edition. Washington, DC, American Psychiatric Association, 1980

American Psychiatric Association: Diagnostic and Statistical Manual of Mental Disorders, 3rd Edition, Revised. Washington, DC, American Psychiatric Association, 1987

Anthony EJ: Neurotic disorders, in Comprehensive Textbook of Psychiatry. Edited by Freedman AM, Kaplan HI, Sadock BJ. Baltimore, MD, Williams & Wilkins, 1975, pp 2143–2160

Cantwell DP, Baker L: Psychiatric and learning disorders in children with speech and language disorders: a descriptive analysis. Advances in Learning and Behavioral Disabilities 4:29–47, 1985

Gittelman R: Childhood anxiety disorders: correlates and outcomes, in Anxiety Disorders of Childhood. Edited by Gittelman R. New York, Guilford, 1986, pp 101–125

Group for the Advancement of Psychiatry: Psychopathological Disorders in Childhood: Theoretical Considerations and a Proposed Classification (GAP Report 62). New York, Group for the Advancement of Psychiatry, 1966

Last CG, Francis G: School phobia, in Advances in Clinical Child Psychology, Vol II. Edited by Lahey B, Kazdin A. New York, Plenum, 1988, pp 193–222

Last CG, Phillips JE, Statfeld A: Childhood anxiety disorders in mothers and their children. Child Psychiatry Hum Dev 18:103–112, 1987a

Last CG, Hersen M, Kazdin AE, et al: Comparison of DSM III separation anxiety and overanxious disorders: demographic characteristics and patterns of co-morbidity. J Am Acad Child Psychiatry 26:527–531, 1987b

Last CG, Hersen M, Kazdin AE, et al: Psychiatric illness in the mothers of anxious children. Am J Psychiatry 12:1580–1583, 1987c

Last CG, Francis G, Hersen M, et al: Separation anxiety and school phobia: a comparison using DSM III criteria. Am J Psychiatry 144:635–657, 1987d

Last CG, Francis G, Strauss CC: Assessing fears in anxiety disordered children with the revised fear survey schedule for children (FSSC-R). J Clin Child Psychol 18:137–141, 1989

Pfohl B, Andreasen NA: Development of classification systems in psychiatry. Compr Psychiatry 19:197–207, 1978

Rutter M: Research report: Institute of Psychiatry Department of Child and Adolescent Psychiatry. Psychol Med 6:505–516, 1976

Rutter M, Tizard J, Yule W, et al: Research report: the Isle of Wight studies, 1964–1974. Psychol Med 6:313–332, 1976

World Health Organization: Manual of International Statistical Classification of Diseases: Injuries and Causes of Death, 5th Revision, Vol I. Geneva, World Health Organization, 1938

World Health Organization: Manual of International Statistical Classification of Diseases: Injuries and Causes of Death, 6th Revision, Vol I. Geneva, World Health Organization, 1948

World Health Organization: Manual of International Statistical Classification of Diseases: Injuries and Causes of Death, 7th Revision, Vol I. Geneva, World Health Organization, 1955

World Health Organization: Manual of International Statistical Classification of Diseases: Injuries and Causes of Death, 8th Revision, Vol I. Geneva, World Health Organization, 1967

World Health Organization: Manual of International Statistical Classification of Diseases: Injuries and Causes of Death, 9th Revision, Vol I. Geneva, World Health Organization, 1975

World Health Organization: Mental behavioral and developmental disorders (Chapter V [F]), in Manual of International Statistical Classification of Diseases, 10th Revision. 1986 Draft for Field Trials. Geneva, World Health Organization, 1987, pp 152–171

Chapter 6

Separation Anxiety Disorder

*I*t has been well known since antiquity that children are particularly sensitive to threats of abandonment and separation by their caregivers and worry about not being adequately protected or cared for. The themes of many fairy tales reflect characteristics of separation anxiety that are forever abolished at their conclusion when the person is rescued and reunited with those who provide protection, consolation, and lasting security.

Normal developmental separation anxiety begins to manifest itself in children around 6 to 8 months of age when infants start to recognize their caregivers and develop an emotional bond or attachment with them. The development of this bond serves the biological function of primary protection of the infant from harm. This relationship instills in the infant a basic sense of trust and lays the foundation for later relationships. Similarly, the separation anxiety that develops within this adaptive relationship serves as the prototype for later anxiety.

The attachment theory contends that separation anxiety is a primary instinctual system that has evolved in order to establish close social bonds and to make maternal or other caregiver separation precipitate anxiety, thus ensuring survival.

Bowlby (1973) has described three stages of emotional reactions in children who are separated from their caregivers on a temporary basis. These include "protest," "despair," and "detachment." On separation the child lodges a protest by screaming and throwing a fit in the presence of the departing parent. This stage of protest may begin immediately or may be delayed; its duration ranges from a few hours to a week (or more) after the caregiver has left. During this period the child is acutely distressed, engages in searching behavior to locate his or her mother, and exhibits motor and vocal agitation. The child tends to reject any consolation or support, although he or she may cling to the baby-sitter. This stage is followed by a period of despair during which the child shows signs of anxiety, worry, and increasing hopelessness. The motor and vocal agitation diminishes, although the child may cry intermittently and appear to be in a state of deep mourning. Comfort and consolation provided by the substitute caregiver eventually help the child settle down and become involved in other activities. The third stage, "detachment," occurs on the parent's return when the child shows little, if any, excitement at the reunion.

A more severe form of reaction to separation from the caregiver is described by Spitz and Wolf (1946) as "anaclitic depression." In their study, 19 of 123 infants observed between 12 and 18 months of age developed a "weepy" behavior that contrasted markedly with their previously happy and outgoing predisposition. After a time this weepiness gave way to withdrawal. For example, they would lie in their cots with averted faces, refusing to take part in their surroundings. Spitz and Wolf attributed this syndrome to the infants being separated from their mothers (or loved object). In all cases, when the mother was reunited with the child following a separation of 3 or 4 months, the anaclitic depression disappeared.

There are many other examples of minor anxiety symptoms in childhood that are normal and transient. When these symptoms are severe enough to cause dysfunction and distress, the condition should be considered a disorder.

Separation anxiety disorder has been discussed in the earlier literature, usually in relation to school phobia. Most authors have supported its existence. Johnson and her colleagues (1941), who first coined the term "school phobia," attributed this condition to an underlying hostile and dependent relationship between child and mother with the child's consequent dread of separation from her. Later these same workers (Estes et al. 1956) replaced the term school phobia with "separation anxiety disorder" in order to emphasize the underlying psychopathology and to remove confusion created by the former term.

Bowlby (1973), in discussing "separation anxiety and anger," attributed school phobia in a child to his or her fear of absence or loss of an attachment figure (i.e., mother) or a security base (i.e., home). Bowlby's theory was later incorporated into the DSM-III diagnosis of separation anxiety disorder, the essential feature of which was excessive anxiety concerning separation from a major attachment figure or home (American Psychiatric Association 1980). Very little empirical research addressing separation anxiety disorder in children and adolescents predated DSM-III. Since this revision, however, a number of reports have appeared in the literature that have addressed some aspect of anxiety disorder (Bernstein and Garfinkel 1986; Cantwell and Baker 1989; Hershberg et al. 1982; Last et al. 1987a, 1987b, 1987c, 1987d). These studies support the notion that separation anxiety disorder is a distinct psychiatric entity. Most authors agree that the diagnostic criteria for anxiety disorders need further refinement in order to prevent overlap.

Definition of Separation Anxiety Disorder (SAD)

SAD is defined as excessive, persistent, and unrealistic worry about separation from either the mother or primary attachment figure to the extent that the anxiety symptoms are very painful and cause a significant impairment or disability in one or more important areas of the child's functioning.

Gittelman-Klein (1988) identifies three characteristics of SAD. First, the distress produced by separation from the mother is very severe and may approach a panic state in its most severe form. Second, a number of morbid worries about potential dangers threatening one or more members of the family must be present. Third, there must be an intense desire for reunification with family or home to a degree that transcends common homesickness.

Epidemiology

The epidemiology of anxiety disorders in general has been discussed in detail in Chapter 3. As pointed out earlier, most of these studies preceded DSM-III and most reported global estimates of maladjustment rather than estimates of specific disorders (Schwartz-Gould et al. 1981). Early studies that focused on specific conditions suffered from a number of methodological problems. They utilized various methods of assessment, criteria, and informants (Orvaschel and Weissman 1986), and the data were limited to symptoms prevalence estimates.

Another set of reports providing data on the prevalence of SAD in children includes studies of school phobia and agoraphobia in adults. It is estimated by some authors that as many as 80% of children diagnosed with school phobia actually suffer from SAD (Gittelman and Klein 1984). SAD was also found in the childhood history of 50% of adults diagnosed with agoraphobia (Gittelman and Klein 1984).

More and more researchers routinely use DSM-III criteria and standardized measurement to study SAD and other anxiety disorders. Anderson et al. (1987) studied 792 11-year-old children from the general New Zealand population using structured child interviews and standardized parent and teacher questionnaires. He found a 1-year prevalence rate of SAD of 3.5%. Females were overrepresented in all anxiety disorders except overanxious disorder.

In another study (Weissman et al. 1984) the authors examined the prevalence of SAD in 6- to 8-year-old children of depressed and normal adults. They used DSM-III diagnostic criteria and relied on direct structured clinical interviews to establish the diagnosis. The depressed parents were separated into four different clinical groups: those without any anxiety disorder and those with agoraphobia, panic disorder, or generalized anxiety disorder. SAD was diagnosed in 24% of children whose parents had a diagnosis of both depression and agoraphobia but in only 6% of children whose parents had depression and generalized anxiety disorder. In a more recent and comprehensive demographic study using DSM-III criteria (Last et al. 1987b), 91 children were evaluated at a child and adolescent anxiety disorder clinic (age range 5–18 years) from September 1984 through February 1986. Of those 91 children, 22 (24%) were found to have SAD. Of these, 64% were female, 91% were under 13 years of age, and 86% were white. According to the Hollingshead index, 75% were rated below socioeconomic status IV and V.

Another study reported by Cantwell and Baker (1980, 1985, 1988) involved 151 children aged 2.3 to 15.9 years (mean age = 5.9 years; SD = 2.9 years) who had some impairment in speech or language functioning, or both (disorder of speech production = 23%, disorder of both speech and language = 65%, and disorder of language development = 12%) but who had normal intelligence. Psychiatric diagnosis was based on DSM-III diagnostic criteria employing four types of instruments: parent and child interviews (Diagnostic Interview for Child and Adolescents and Diagnostic Interview for Child and Adolescents, Parents' Version) (Orvaschel 1985) and parent and teacher behavior rating scales (two forms for each) (Conners 1973; Rutter et al. 1970). Of the 151 children, 21% (n = 31) had anxiety disorders and 6% (n = 9) had SAD. The age of these children ranged from 2.4 to 6.6 years (mean age = 3.6 years; SD = 1.3 years), and 56% were boys. Bird et al. (1988) carried out a two-stage epidemiological survey of 4- to

16-year-old Puerto Rican children using a screening instrument and the child behavior checklist. A diagnosis of SAD was made in 4.7% (weighted percentage) of the children; frequency of the disorder peaked in the 6- to 11-year-old age group.

Clinical Features

The key clinical feature of SAD is a focused excessive anxiety concerning separation from those individuals to whom the child is attached—usually parents or another family member. This anxiety may approach the level of panic in intensity and may be manifested in many different forms. Often these children report an unrealistic preoccupying worry about the welfare of their parents or siblings. Afraid that harm may come to this caregiver during their absence, these children may lodge strong protest around the time of the caregiver's departure for work or grocery shopping. They are also fearful that a parent may leave and never return, or that some untoward event such as being lost or kidnapped will separate them from the parent.

Many children suffering from SAD refuse to go to school, not because of any deterrent per se at school, but rather because of what might happen to their parents during the child's absence. Often they report preoccupation with thoughts of their parents while in the classroom. Last et al. (1987d) found that approximately three-quarters of children who met the DSM-III criteria for separation anxiety also showed avoidance of or reluctance to go to school. SAD children avoid visiting friends, traveling independently, or even going alone from room to room or into a vacant room in their own home. These children show clinging behavior, frequently "shadowing" their parents at home. They refuse to be alone in their home and demand the presence of a parent or a family member in the house at all times. These children are either persistently reluctant or simply refuse to sleep alone without being next to a parent or family member. SAD children may have frequent nightmares with separation themes, often resulting in reluctance to go to sleep.

Somatic complaints are frequently encountered in SAD children. These symptoms are reported either in anticipation or at the time of separation. The child may persistently complain of abdominal pain, nausea, or headaches every Monday morning or after a holiday break.

Moreover, monsters, animal fears, and death phobia (of self and of loved ones) are commonly reported by SAD children.

Older children and adolescents may present a slightly different clinical picture. For example, adolescents more often demonstrate anticipatory anxiety toward potential identifiable dangers such as the father dying during an airplane trip. These patients may deny their fear of separation or of parental danger, but their behavior clearly reflects their morbid anxiety and fear. Older children and adolescents may also complain more frequently of cardiovascular symptoms such as palpitations, chest pains, and choking or smothering sensations.

Age at Onset

By definition, the age at onset is before 18 years (American Psychiatric Association 1987); however, it may begin as early as the preschool years. In Cantwell and Baker's study (1989) the age of children diagnosed with SAD by DSM-III criteria ($n = 9$) ranged from 2.4 to 6.6 years (mean = 3.6 years; SD = 1.3 years). The children with SAD reported by Last et al. (1987b) were relatively older at the time of the evaluation ($n = 48$; mean age = 9.4 years; SD = 2.9).

Associated features of SAD may include a variety of fears, particularly of the dark. Children may insist on leaving the bedroom light on at night, and they may attribute their discomfort to "seeing" or "feeling" eyes staring at them in the dark or to mythical animals or bloody creatures "ganging up" on them. SAD children may look sad and report feeling depressed. They cry easily and sometimes complain of not being loved or that their siblings are favored over them. They may express wishes to die. Parents frequently describe these children as demanding and wanting constant attention.

Diagnosis

The general principles of and assessment tools used for diagnosis are discussed at length in Chapter 4 and will be discussed briefly herein.

DSM-III-R Criteria for Diagnosis of SAD

The specific diagnostic criteria used by DSM-III-R are generally accepted for clinical purposes and include the following:

A. Excessive anxiety concerning separation from those to whom the child is attached, as evidenced by at least three of the following:
 1. Unrealistic and persistent worry about possible harm befalling major attachment figures or fear that they will leave and not return.
 2. Unrealistic and persistent worry that an untoward calamitous event will separate the child from a major attachment figure, e.g., the child will be lost, kidnapped, killed, or the victim of an accident.
 3. Persistent reluctance or refusal to go to school in order to stay with major attachment figures or at home.
 4. Persistent reluctance or refusal to go to sleep without being near a major attachment figure or to go to sleep away from home.
 5. Persistent avoidance of being alone, including "clinging to" and "shadowing" major attachment figures.
 6. Repeated nightmares involving the theme of separation.
 7. Complaints of physical symptoms, e.g., headaches, stomachaches, nausea, or vomiting, on many school days or on other occasions when anticipating separation from major attachment figures.
 8. Recurrent signs or complaints of excessive distress in anticipation of separation from home or major attachment figures, e.g., temper tantrums or crying, pleading with parents not to leave.
 9. Recurrent signs or complaints of excessive distress when separated from home or major attachment figures, e.g., wants to return home or needs to call parents when they are absent or when child is away from home.
B. Duration of disturbance of at least 2 weeks.
C. Onset before age 18 years.
D. Occurrence not exclusively during the course of a pervasive developmental disorder, schizophrenia, or any other psychotic disorder.

Differential Diagnosis

It is normal for young children to show some anxiety over real or threatened separation from their parents or those to whom they are primarily attached. SAD should be distinguished from developmentally appropriate separation anxiety. Even when the child shows abnormally persistent anxiety beyond the usual age period and with associated impaired social functioning, SAD should not be diagnosed if symptoms are due to a pervasive developmental disorder, schizophrenia, or any other psychotic disorder. Similarly, with a diagnosis of overanxious disorder, avoidant disorder of childhood or adolescence, conduct disorder with school refusal, or phobic disorder, the diagnosis of SAD should be excluded. SAD may be considered either a primary or a secondary diagnosis in the case of hyperactivity, minimal brain dysfunction, or enuresis. In major depression occurring during childhood, the diagnosis of separation anxiety should also be made only when the criteria for both disorders are met (American Psychiatric Association 1987).

Natural History

Follow-up studies on children with SAD mostly predate the DSM-III era and primarily describe the course and prognosis of children with school refusals (Berg 1976; Berg and Fielding 1978; Berg and Jackson 1985; Waldron 1976). Berg and Jackson (1985) studied 168 school refusers 10 years after their discharge from a treatment facility and identified predictors of favorable outcome. They found high intelligence level, treatment intervention before 14 years of age, and symptom remission prior to initial treatment intervention to correlate well with a good prognosis.

More recently Cantwell and Baker studied the stability of DSM-III childhood diagnoses (Cantwell and Baker 1989). They conducted psychiatric evaluation of 151 children on referral of the children to a community speech and language clinic and again approximately 4 years later, using DSM-III criteria. The follow-up psychiatric diagnoses were made "semiblind" to the initial psychiatric diagnosis. Nine children were diagnosed as having pure SAD on initial evaluation. Four years later four of these children (44% of the group) were well. SAD persisted in only one child. Two children had behavior disorders (attention-deficit disorder with hyperactivity and attention-deficit disorder without hyperactivity), and three had overanxious disorder. It is interesting to note that one child with SAD initially had comorbid diagnoses of attention-deficit disorder without hyperactivity and overanxious disorder at follow-up. The authors concluded that SAD was relatively more unstable than other DSM-III anxiety disorders. They attributed some of this instability to the very young age of this group (mean age = 3.6 years; SD = 1.3).

In summary, the natural course of SAD generally consists of waxing and waning symptomatology that may fluctuate over several years. Alternately, SAD may also remit spontaneously after one episode. Exacerbation may also occur in adolescence or young adulthood when a person is faced with situations such as leaving home for college or geographic relocation to a new job (Werkman 1987). Some authors (Gittelman and Klein 1984) have reported that SAD predisposes children to the development of agoraphobia in adult life. Others (Coolidge et al. 1964) suggest that children with school phobia and probable underlying SAD are more likely to develop work phobia later in life.

Treatment

The treatment of childhood anxiety disorder is discussed in more detail in Chapter 12. Only the specific treatment of SAD will be briefly discussed here.

Three treatment modalities—pharmacotherapy (Gittelman and Koplewicz 1986), behavior therapy (Carlson et al. 1986), and psychodynamically oriented psychotherapy (Lewis 1986), either alone or in combination—have been found to be effective in the treatment of SAD.

Many mild cases of separation anxiety with school phobia are effectively handled by a combination of emotional support for the child and the parent (usually the mother) along with coercion of the child to return to school.

A combination of dynamically oriented psychotherapy and behavior therapy techniques for the child and the family has been proven to be most effective for more severe forms of this disorder. Both implosion and systematic desensitization have been successful in returning the child to school and reducing separation anxiety.

Behavior modification techniques may also be employed to teach the child relaxation techniques. This may involve the use of progressive gradual desensitization procedures for specific causes of anxiety.

Gittelman-Klein and Klein (1971) found imipramine in combination with behavior modification to be successful in treating panic attacks in children with SAD. Other antianxiety medications such as the benzodiazepines have also been shown to temporarily alleviate the symptoms of anxiety.

As a last resort, children may benefit from admission to a psychiatric inpatient or day treatment program when a dysfunctional home or family situation is reinforcing the child's anxiety.

References

American Psychiatric Association: Diagnostic and Statistical Manual of Mental Disorders, 3rd Edition. Washington, DC, American Psychiatric Association, 1980

American Psychiatric Association: Diagnostic and Statistical Manual of Mental Disorders, 3rd Edition, Revised. Washington, DC, American Psychiatric Association, 1987

Anderson JC, William S, McGee R, et al: DSM-III disorders in preadolescent children. Arch Gen Psychiatry 44:69–76, 1987

Berg I: School phobia in children of agoraphobic women. Br J Psychiatry 128:86–89, 1976

Berg I, Fielding D: An evaluation of hospital inpatient treatment in adolescent school phobia. Br J Psychiatry 132:500–505, 1978

Berg I, Jackson A: Teenage school refusers grow up: a follow-up study of 168 subjects, ten years on average after inpatient treatment. Br J Psychiatry 47:366–370, 1985

Bernstein GA, Garfinkel B: School phobia: the overlap of affective and anxiety disorders. J Am Acad Child Psychiatry 25:235–241, 1986

Bird HR, Canino G, Rubio-Stipec M, et al: Estimates of the prevalence of childhood maladjustment in a community survey in Puerto Rico. Arch Gen Psychiatry 45:1120–1126, 1988

Bowlby J: Separation: Anxiety and Anger (Attachment and Loss Series, Vol 2). New York, Basic Books, 1973

Cantwell DP, Baker L: Psychiatric and behavioral characteristics of children with communication disorders. J Pediatr Psychol 5:161–178, 1980

Cantwell DP, Baker L: Psychiatric and learning disorders in children with speech and language disorders: a descriptive analysis. Advances in Learning and Behavioral Disabilities 4:29–47, 1985

Cantwell DP, Baker L: Anxiety disorders in children with communication disorders. Journal of Anxiety Disorders 2:135–146, 1988

Cantwell DP, Baker L: Stability and natural history of DSM-III childhood diagnoses. J Am Acad Child Adolesc Psychiatry 28(5):691–700, 1989

Carlson CL, Figueroa RG, Lahey BB: Behavior therapy for childhood anxiety disorders, in Anxiety Disorders of Childhood. Edited by Gittelman R. New York, Guilford, 1986, pp 204–232

Conners CK: Rating scales for use in drug studies with children. Psychopharmacol Bull (special issue), 1973, pp 24–34

Coolidge JC, Brodie RD, Feeney B: A ten year follow up study of sixty six school children. Am J Orthopsychiatry 34:675–684, 1964

Estes H, Haylet E, Johnson E: Separation anxiety. Am J Psychotherapy 10:682–695, 1956

Gittelman R, Klein DF: Relationship between separation anxiety and panic and agoraphobic disorders. Psychopathology 17 (suppl 1):56–65, 1984

Gittelman R, Koplewicz HS: Pharmacotherapy of childhood anxiety disorders, in Anxiety Disorders of Childhood. Edited by Gittelman R. New York, Guilford, 1986, pp 188–203

Gittelman-Klein R: Childhood anxiety disorders, in Handbook of Clinical Assessment of Children and Adolescents, Vol II. Edited by Kestenbaum CJ, Williams DT. New York, New York University Press, 1988, pp 722–742

Gittelman-Klein R, Klein DF: Controlled imipramine treatment of school phobia. Arch Gen Psychiatry 25:204–207, 1971

Hershberg SG, Carlson GA, Cantwell DP, et al: Anxiety and depressive disorders in psychiatrically disturbed children. J Clin Psychiatry 43:358–361, 1982

Johnson A, Folstein E, Stanislaus A, et al: School phobia. Am J Orthopsychiatry 11:702–711, 1941

Last CG, Phillips JE, Statfeld A: Childhood anxiety disorders in mothers and their children. Child Psychiatry Hum Dev 18:103–112, 1987a

Last CG, Hersen M, Kazdin AE, et al: Comparison of DSM-III separation anxiety and overanxious disorders: demographic characteristics and patterns of comorbidity. J Am Acad Child Psychiatry 26:527–531, 1987b

Last CG, Hersen M, Kazdin AE, et al: Psychiatric illness in the mothers of anxious children. Am J Psychiatry 12:1580–1583, 1987c

Last CG, Francis G, Hersen M, et al: Separation anxiety and school phobia: a comparison using DSM-III criteria. Am J Psychiatry 144:635–657, 1987d

Lewis M: Principles of intensive individual psychoanalytic psychotherapy for childhood anxiety disorders, in Anxiety Disorders of Childhood. Edited by Gittelman R. New York, Guilford, 1986, pp 233–256

Orvaschel H: Psychiatric interviews suitable for use in research with children and adolescents. Psychopharmacol Bull 21:737–746, 1985

Orvaschel H, Weissman MM: Epidemiology of anxiety disorders in children: a review, in Anxiety Disorders of Childhood. Edited by Gittelman R. New York, Guilford, 1986, pp 58–72

Rutter M, Tizard J, Whitmore K: Education, Health and Behavior. London, Longman, 1970

Schwartz-Gould M, Wunsch-Hitzig R, Dohrenwend B: Estimating the prevalence of childhood psychopathology: a critical review. J Am Acad Child Psychiatry 20:462–476, 1981

Spitz RA, Wolf KM: The smiling response: a contribution to the ontogenesis of social relations. Genetic Psychology Monographs 34:57–125, 1946

Waldron S: The significance of childhood neurosis for adult mental health: a follow up study. Am J Psychiatry 133:532–538, 1976

Weissman MM, Leckman JR, Merikangar KR, et al: Depression and anxiety disorders in parents and children: results from the Yale Family Study. Arch Gen Psychiatry 41:845–852, 1984

Werkman S: Anxiety disorders, in Comprehensive Textbook of Psychiatry, Vol III. Edited by Kaplan HI, Freedman AM, Sadock BJ. Baltimore, MD, Williams & Wilkins, 1987, pp 2620–2631

Chapter 7

Avoidant Disorder of Childhood or Adolescence

*U*nlike separation anxiety disorder, very little attention has been paid to avoidant disorder of childhood or adolescence; it appears for the first time in DSM-III (American Psychiatric Association 1980). In DSM-II (American Psychiatric Association 1968) a condition with "withdrawing reaction" was described under the broader category of "behavior disorders of childhood and adolescence" and was characterized by "seclusiveness, detachment, sensitivity, timidity, and general inability to form close interpersonal relationships" (p. 50). Although some characteristics of avoiding reaction are also listed for avoidant disorder, the key difference between the two is that in avoidant disorder withdrawal is from unfamiliar people, while a desire for contact with familiar people, such as family members, is maintained (American Psychiatric Association 1987).

Although DSM-III has been criticized for its categories (Quay 1987; Rutter and Shaffer 1980), one of the arguments in support of its classification of childhood anxiety disorders is that each disorder can be related to stages of development or age-specific types of anxiety (Werry and Aman 1980). For example, overanxious disorder can be viewed as an exaggeration of elemental anxiety present at birth; avoidant disorder can be viewed as the continuation of stranger anxiety; and so on.

It is now well documented from a number of studies that infants begin to markedly alter their responses to strangeness around 8 months of age (Emde et al. 1976; Harmon et al. 1977; Sroufe 1977). Before 5–6 months of age, infants show no avoidance behavior when they encounter unfamiliarity alone. As they grow older, they begin to show worry by frowning, worried facies, gaze aversion, and cardiac acceleration. Impulsivity toward an unfamiliar object diminishes, and they also become very cautious in reaching for strange objects. These behavioral responses toward strangers evolve, too. These age-dependent trends are observed across cultures (Goldberg 1972; Konner 1972) and have been found to be less frequent at home or with the mother than in the laboratory (Kagan 1974; Skarin 1977; Sroufe et al. 1974).

Another area of research concerning avoidant disorder involves primary behavior patterns or temperaments. It is now agreed that individual behavioral differences exist from birth. These differences were first systematically observed by Thomas et al. (1963), who factor-analyzed nine primary temperament parameters in children. These include activity level; regularity of biological functions such as sleep, hunger, and elimination; approach and withdrawal from new situations, including persons, places, foods, etc.; adaptability to new situations; threshold of responsiveness; quality of mood; intensity of emotional reaction; distractibility; and attention span. These differences influence the way children respond to their environment as well as how their parents and others react to them. Based on combinations of these parameters, Chess et al. (1965) divided children on the basis of the following scheme: the "easy to warm up" child, the "difficult" child, and the "slow to warm up" child. Only the last is relevant to our discussion of avoidant disorder. This child has a low activity level, has an initial withdrawal response to new situations, adapts poorly to unfamiliar people and circumstances, and may be predisposed to future avoidant disorder (Rutter et al. 1964).

Epidemiology

A comprehensive discussion of the epidemiology of anxiety disorders is found in Chapter 3. As mentioned earlier, avoidant disorder as a separate category was not listed until DSM-III. Only a few studies have reported on the demographics of avoidant disorder in the clinic population, and no data as yet are available on the prevalence of anxiety disorder in the general population.

Cantwell and Baker (1989) reported on a follow-up study of children who initially had a psychiatric diagnosis by DSM-III criteria and who were referred for speech and language evaluation. Of the 151 children, 31 (20.5%) met the DSM-III criteria for an anxiety disorder, with avoidant disorder being the most prevalent subgroup ($n = 14$, 9.3%). The children ranged in age from 3.1 years to 9.7 years (mean = 5.0; SD = 1.9) and consisted of eight girls and six boys.

In another study of children referred to an anxiety clinic over a 24-month period, Francis and colleagues collected information on 22 children with avoidant disorder (G. Francis, C.G. Last, C.C. Strauss, unpublished data, 1988). Their data suggest that avoidant disorder can occur at any age, with a mean age of 12.7 years and with an equal incidence rate below and above 13 years of age. Sixteen (73%) were females and 94% were Caucasian. The socioeconomic status was divided equally between upper and lower strata. These authors suggest that avoidant disorder is less common than either separation anxiety disorder or overanxious disorder, and rarely occurs alone. In their study, almost every child with avoidant disorder had an additional concurrent anxiety disorder diagnosis, most commonly overanxious disorder. The higher incidence of avoidant disorder found by Cantwell and Baker (1989) may be explained in terms of the population studied. Self-consciousness among these children with speech and language disorder may well have predisposed them to avoidance of unfamiliar people.

Clinical Features

In clinical practice avoidant disorder is encountered more frequently in girls than in boys. Children with this disorder demonstrate an excessive resistance to contact with unfamiliar children and adults. This holding-back behavior is severe enough to cause impaired, dysfunctional interpersonal relationships. This avoidance of strangers persists in spite of prolonged and repeated exposure to strangers. Conversely, these children desire close contact with family members and indulge them with warm and affectionate interaction.

In the presence of an unfamiliar person, children with avoidant disorder appear socially withdrawn, embarrassed, and timid; they speak in a low-toned whisper in an attempt to remain inconspicuous. Their discomfort becomes more pronounced and at times may erupt into anger when prodded by parents to socialize and interact with strangers. Relationships with peers are virtually nonexistent, and these children seldom complain of not having any friends.

Children with avoidant disorder are seldom brought to the mental health clinic by their parents, who, although aware of their "shyness," do not consider their behavior dysfunctional. Rather, teachers are frequently the first to become concerned about their nonassertive, passive attitude, lack of interaction with peers, and refusal to participate in group activities. Their academic performance is generally not hampered except in those subjects requiring exposure to other individuals, such as physical education, where they have to undress in front of peers or compete with them. In fact they often become the target of their peers' ridicule. They are often mistaken as oppositional or defiant and may fall from the grace of their teachers. School experiences become unpleasant for them and school avoidance sometimes follows.

Their conduct during a psychiatric interview is also typical of their behavior in an unfamiliar situation. They are usually anxious and poorly responsive or mute, and hide behind their parents. The more they are pressed to respond, the more they wither and retreat. Those clinicians who recognize the condition of these children early and spare them from vigorous interrogation fare better with them in the long run. Much more yardage is gained by working with these children through their parents.

Often these children reveal a self-critical attitude and demand perfection from themselves. Consequently, they shy away from competition. They may confide to their parents or therapist about grandiose fantasies of unrecognized capabilities and complain of not receiving due recognition. They also may share with them tales of imaginary companions.

Diagnosis and Assessment

The general principles of diagnosis and the assessment tools for anxiety disorders are discussed in Chapter 4. Only those DSM-III-R diagnostic criteria specific to avoidant disorder will be discussed here briefly.

A. Excessive shrinking from contact with unfamiliar people, for a period of 6 months or longer, sufficiently severe to interfere with social functioning in peer relationships.
B. Desire for social involvement with familiar people (family members and peers the person knows well) and generally warm and satisfying relations with family members and other familiar figures.
C. Age at least 2½ years.
D. The disturbance is not sufficiently pervasive and persistent to warrant the diagnosis of avoidant personality disorder.

Differential Diagnosis

Avoidant disorder should be differentiated from stranger anxiety, which is normally present between approximately 8 months and 2½ years of age. Therefore, the diagnosis of avoidant disorder should not be made in children younger than 2½ years. In socially reticent and "slow to warm up" children, some degree of adaptability occurs after a short period of time. They often hang around the periphery of a peer group, slowly approaching and finally integrating with them. In children with avoidant disorder, the adaptability to new and unfamiliar people is almost nonexistent.

Avoidant disorder should also be distinguished from separation anxiety disorder and overanxious disorder. In separation anxiety disorder the focus is on separation from a parent or a major attachment figure rather than avoidance of an unfamiliar person. It is important to note, however, that according to some authors avoidant disorder frequently coexists with separation anxiety disorder or overanxious disorder (G. Francis, C.G. Last, C.C. Strauss, unpublished data, 1988). In overanxious disorder the anxiety is more generalized and unrelated to unfamiliar figures.

Children with schizoid disorder are distinguished by more severe character pathology and more intense and diffuse symptomatology. They are withdrawn from everyone, including their parents. These children are generally distant, and unlike children with avoidant disorder, they are incapable of developing warm and loving relationships with family members. They do not enjoy peer relationships and are altogether socially detached.

Avoidant disorder may also be confused with an adjustment disorder in which withdrawal is related to a recent psychosocial stress and is not chronic in its course.

Patients with an avoidant disorder personality are usually older (18 years or more), and symptoms have usually been present for several years.

Natural History

Avoidant disorder is probably the most stable of the childhood anxiety disorders. In Cantwell and Baker's (1989) follow-up study, only 4 of 14 children (29%) initially diagnosed as having avoidant disorder still had the same diagnosis 4 years later. Most (64%), however, remained psychiatrically ill. Four of the children initially diagnosed with avoidant disorder had overanxious disorder at follow-up, and 2 had dysthymic disorder.

Though the natural course of avoidant disorder requires much greater study, the preliminary data indicate a chronic course. The failure of a child to establish social contacts outside the family may lead to feelings of isolation and depression. The personality traits that characterize avoidant disorder may, on the other hand, eventuate in schizoid or borderline personality structures; the progression to avoidant personality disorder in adulthood is probably rare.

If left untreated, many children with avoidant disorder will recover spontaneously. This is more likely to occur after a positive social experience with peers, such as becoming an active member of a social group.

Treatment

General and specific treatment modalities for childhood anxiety disorders are discussed in detail in Chapter 12, and treatment will be discussed briefly here. Very little current literature is available on the treatment of avoidant disorder. A number of treatment modalities have been utilized, including play therapy, behavior modification, cognitive therapy, family therapy, and psychopharmacotherapy.

Noncorrective play therapy has been shown to be most effective in younger children whose home environment is fairly restrictive (Axline 1964). By developing a relationship with the child, the therapist helps him or her to overcome social inhibition while simultaneously increasing his or her self-confidence and assertiveness. The teaching of such skills as dancing, singing, or writing may serve to enhance much-needed ego support.

A variety of behavioral programs have described the successful emergence of children with avoidant disorder from social isolation. Ross (1970) used modeling with guided participation, in which the therapist would lead the child through tasks that were previously shunned due to fear. The tasks were arranged in a hierarchy of difficulty, with the therapist first demonstrating them and then participating with the child in that activity. Eventually the child's success was signaled by performing the feared task alone (Ross 1970). Teachers' use of social reinforcers and social skills training by videotape have also been found to be effective in modifying isolated behavior (Schaefer and Millman 1977).

Family therapy may become necessary when the parents and other family members consciously or unconsciously reinforce the child's dependency and isolation behavior. Sometimes such parental reinforcement may actually indicate an underlying depression in the parents. Accordingly, treatment for the parent as well as the child is warranted.

In contrast to separation anxiety disorder, the use of antianxiety or sedative drugs is seldom indicated in avoidant disorder. Medications of this type would merely reinforce passivity and withdrawal, and would undermine the goal of therapy, i.e., to help the child master his or her anxiety in order to gain a higher degree of independent functioning. Psychopharmacotherapy may become necessary, however, when concurrent conditions (e.g., overanxious disorder or depression) exist. In such cases an appropriate antidepressant or anxiolytic agent may prove to be an adjunct to other therapies.

Moreover, social phobias in adults, which may be viewed as the developmental variant of childhood avoidant disorder, have been successfully treated with phenelzine, a monoamine oxidase inhibitor (Liebowitz et al. 1986).

References

American Psychiatric Association: Diagnostic and Statistical Manual of Mental Disorders, 2nd Edition. Washington, DC, American Psychiatric Association, 1968

American Psychiatric Association: Diagnostic and Statistical Manual of Mental Disorders, 3rd Edition. Washington, DC, American Psychiatric Association, 1980

American Psychiatric Association: Diagnostic and Statistical Manual of Mental Disorders, 3rd Edition, Revised. Washington, DC, American Psychiatric Association, 1987

Axline VM: Non-directive therapy, in Child Psychotherapy. Edited by Haworth MR. New York, Basic Books, 1964, pp 34–39

Cantwell DP, Baker L: Stability and natural history of DSM III childhood diagnoses. J Am Acad Child Adolesc Psychiatry 28(5):691–700, 1989

Chess S, Thomas A, Birch H: Your Child Is a Person. New York, Penguin, 1965

Emde RN, Gaensbauer TJ, Harmon RJ: Emotional Expression in Infancy. New York, International Universities Press, 1976

Goldberg S: Infant care and growth in urban Zambia. Hum Dev 15:77–89, 1972

Harmon R, Morgan G, Klein R: Determinant of normal variation in infants' negative reactions to unfamiliar adults. J Am Acad Child Psychiatry 16:670–683, 1977

Kagan J: Discrepancy, temperament and infant distress, in The Origins of Fear. Edited by Lewis M, Rosenblum LA. New York, John Wiley, 1974, pp 229–248

Konner M: Aspects of the developmental etiology of a foraging people, in Ethological Studies of Child Behavior. Edited by Blurton Jones N. Cambridge, University of Cambridge Press, 1972

Liebowitz MR, Fyer AJ, Gorman JM, et al: Phenelzine in social phobia. J Clin Psychopharmacol 6:93–98, 1986

Quay HC: A critical analysis of DSM-III as a taxonomy of psychopathology in childhood and adolescence, in Contemporary Issues in Psychopathology. Edited by Millon T, Klerman G. New York, Guilford, 1987

Ross D: Effect on learning of psychological attachment to a film model. Am J Mental Defic 74:701–707, 1970

Rutter M, Shaffer D: DSM-III as step forward or back in terms of classification of child psychiatric disorders. J Am Acad Child Psychiatry 19:371–394, 1980

Rutter M, Birch H, Thomas A, et al: Temperamental characteristics in infancy and later development of behavior disorders. Br J Psychiatry 110:651–661, 1964

Schaefer CE, Millman HI: Therapies for Children. San Francisco, CA, Jossey-Bass, 1977

Skarin K: Cognitive and contextual determinant of stranger fear in 6 and 11 month old infants. Child Dev 48:537–544, 1977

Sroufe LA: Wariness and the study of infant development. Child Dev 48:731–746, 1977

Sroufe LA, Waters E, Matas L: Contextual determinants of infant affective response, in The Origins of Fear. Edited by Lewis M, Rosenblum LA. New York, John Wiley, 1974, pp 49–72

Thomas A, Chess S, Birch H, et al: Behavioral Individuality in Early Childhood. New York, New York University Press, 1963

Werry JS, Aman MG: Anxiety in children, in Handbook of Studies on Anxiety. Edited by Barrows GD, Davies B. Amsterdam, Elsevier North-Holland, 1980

Chapter 8

Overanxious Disorder

Overanxious disorder (OAD) in children has been reported for decades. However, very little empirical research data supporting this diagnosis have been published, even though "overanxious reaction" was one of the first childhood psychiatric conditions included in the DSM system. Based on the clinical studies of Jenkins and Hewitt (1944), this condition was first included in DSM-II (American Psychiatric Association 1968) under the broader category of "behavior disorders of childhood and adolescence." This disorder was characterized by "chronic anxiety, excessive and unrealistic fears, sleeplessness, nightmares and exaggerated autonomic responses. The patient tends to be immature, self-conscious, grossly lacking in self-confidence, conforming, inhibited, dutiful, approval seeking and apprehensive in new situations and unfamiliar surroundings" (American Psychiatric Association 1968, p. 50).

Jenkins and Hewitt (1944) originally attributed these impairments and increased anxiety to a "hypertrophic zone of inhibition (super-ego)" in the child whose parents were demanding, impossible to please, and excessively critical. Under such circumstances the child soon recognized that parental acceptance and approval required control and containment of all primitive impulses (or id drives), even those deemed acceptable (ego syntonic). This situation eventuated in heightened intrapsychic tension and produced a state of chronic anxiety accompanied by nightmares, sleep disturbances, and psychosomatic symptoms.

By the time preparations for DSM-III (American Psychiatric Association 1980) had been completed, sufficient clinical and anecdotal data had become available to permit further subclassification of childhood anxiety disorders. A concept utilized in the formulation of DSM-III was that if a disorder that began regularly in infancy, childhood, or adolescence seemed to resemble another disorder appearing in later life, but differed according to the phenomenology of childhood, then it was listed as a separate disorder with a unique title. In such cases the distinct clinical pictures identified in infancy, childhood, and adolescence were presented. Hence came the inception of a distinct generalized anxiety disorder occurring in childhood, with a slightly different clinical picture from that seen in adults. Further, some developmental theorists conceptualize OAD as an exaggeration of normal elemental anxiety present at birth.

Since the publication of DSM-III, several studies (Bernstein and Garfinkel 1986; Cantwell and Baker 1980, 1985, 1989; Hershberg et al. 1982; Last et al. 1987) have provided data that further support the various categories of anxiety disorders in children. For example, Last et al. (1987) compared the demographic and comorbidity characteristics of separation anxiety disorder and OAD in a sample of 69 children and adolescents. They found that the two disorders differed across several dimensions such as age, social class, and the presence of a coexisting anxiety disorder. Cantwell and Baker (1989) found differences between the childhood anxiety disorders in regard to the stability of diagnosis at follow-up 4 years later.

Epidemiology

There are no data available on the prevalence of OAD in the general population. Last et al. (1987) evaluated 69 children during an 18-month period in an anxiety disorder clinic. Twenty-six of the children (mean age = 13½ years) were diagnosed with OAD; additionally, 21 (30.6%) had a concurrent diagnosis of separation anxiety disorder. The male-to-female ratio was the same for both disorders.

In Cantwell and Baker's previously mentioned studies (1980, 1985, 1989) of 151 children referred to a clinic for speech and language evaluation, 31 (20.5%) had a diagnosis of anxiety disorder according to DSM-III criteria at the time of initial evaluation. Of these, 8 (22.8%) had OAD, 9 (29.0%) had separation anxiety disorder, and 14 (46.2%) had a diagnosis of avoidant disorder. They ranged in age from 4 to 11.2 years (mean = 7.3, SD = 2.3); 63% were male.

Clinical Picture

The cardinal feature of OAD is generalized, persistent anxiety unrelated to a specific situation, person, or object. These children have unrealistic worries about future events or past behaviors. They are doubtful about their competence and worry about their academic or athletic performance, or both. They tend to worry in a ruminative fashion about being judged and found inadequate or incompetent. The children with OAD are very self-conscious and are very sensitive to criticism. They require and seek constant reassurance about their appearance, clothes, performance, and responses.

Children with OAD often complain of multiple physical symptoms such as headaches, stomachaches, and sore throat without any underlying organic cause. They may also complain of a lump in the throat, palpitations, dizziness, or chest pain.

Because they are self-conscious and lack confidence, OAD children frequently perceive various people in their lives as overcritical and hard to please. They typically complain of being ignored or "put down" by their peers, teachers, or coaches and may refuse to participate in certain activities because they feel that they will not receive fair treatment.

Because OAD may accompany other childhood anxiety disorders, signs and symptoms of the concurrent disorder may also be present. In the study by Last et al. (1987) of 91 children referred to an anxiety clinic, 21 (23%) met the criteria for both OAD and separation anxiety disorder. The OAD children may refuse to go to school and may show perfectionist tendencies with self-doubt; they may also be excessively conformist, eagerly seeking to please and gain approval.

The OAD children may appear fidgety and demonstrate nervous habits such as nail biting and hair pulling. They may exhibit excessive autonomic activity with sweaty palms, dry mouth, and so forth.

Some OAD children are very talkative as they diligently scan their environment and ask penetrating questions about events. Hence, they may seem unusually intelligent and precocious, when in fact they are projecting their situation to alleviate anxiety. At other times they may refuse help from adults when attempting difficult tasks.

Diagnosis and Assessment

The general principles involved in the diagnosis and assessment of anxiety disorders are discussed in Chapter 4. Only those issues relevant to the specific diagnosis of OAD and the DSM-III-R (American Psychiatric Association 1987) criteria will be discussed here.

OAD is diagnosed when persistent anxiety and worries about both future and current life events increase to the extent that they impair social relationships and school performance. Excessive somatic complaints and psychophysiological disorders are also frequently present.

DSM-III-R Criteria for Diagnosis of OAD

A. Excessive or unrealistic anxiety or worry, for a period of 6 months or longer, as indicated by the frequent occurrence of at least four of the following:
  1. Excessive or unrealistic worry about future events.
  2. Excessive or unrealistic concern about the appropriateness of past behavior.
  3. Excessive or unrealistic concern about competence in one or more areas, e.g., athletic, academic, social.
  4. Somatic complaints, such as headaches or stomachaches, for which no physical basis can be established.
  5. Marked self-consciousness.
  6. Excessive need for reassurance about a variety of concerns.
  7. Marked feelings of tension or inability to relax.
B. If another Axis I disorder is present (e.g., separation anxiety disorder, phobic disorder, obsessive-compulsive disorder), the focus of the symptoms in A is not limited to it. For example, if separation anxiety disorder is present, the symptoms in A are not exclusively related to anxiety about separation. In addition, the disturbance does not occur only during the course of a psychotic disorder or a mood disorder.
C. If 18 or older, does not meet the criteria for generalized anxiety disorder.
D. Occurrence not exclusively during the course of a pervasive developmental disorder, schizophrenia, or any other psychotic disorder.

Differential Diagnosis

OAD should be distinguished from separation anxiety disorder, in which anxiety is related to a specific situation involving separation from a primary attachment figure. In avoidant disorder the anxiety is related to unfamiliar persons, places, or events.

Similarly, when symptoms of anxiety are due to phobic, obsessive-compulsive, depressive, schizophrenic, or pervasive developmental disorder, the diagnosis of OAD should not be made. Many children with attention-deficit disorder show fidgetiness, motor restlessness, and anxiety. Children with attention-deficit hyperactivity disorder have other symptoms such as impulsivity, aggressiveness, low frustration tolerance, and occasionally associated learning disabilities with soft neurological signs. They have poor motivation to perform, and they frequently have concomitant behavior problems and show no concern for the future. OAD children, in contrast, have a strong motivation to perform well and are eager to please their teachers and conform to school rules and regulations.

In adjustment disorder with anxious mood, the onset of anxiety can be traced to a psychosocial stressor. Premorbid adjustment is usually good, and the condition rarely lasts longer than 6 months.

Natural History

Little is known about the natural history of OAD because this category appeared for the first time in DSM-III. One of the few studies, a short-term follow-up by Cantwell and Baker (1989), involved children referred for speech and language evaluation who also met DSM-III criteria for psychiatric disorder. At follow-up 31 children were diagnosed as having anxiety disorder (separation anxiety disorder = 9, avoidant disorder = 14, and OAD = 8). Of the eight OAD children, only two (25%) continued to have OAD at 4-year follow-up. Of all the anxiety disorder subgroups, the overanxious group had the lowest recovery rate. Only two (25%) of the OAD children were psychiatrically well at follow-up. The others had avoidant disorder (two cases), attention-deficit disorder with hyperactivity (one case), attention-deficit disorder without hyperactivity (two cases), and major depression (one case). Two of the OAD children at follow-up had multiple diagnoses (avoidant disorder and OAD in one case; avoidant disorder and attention-deficit disorder without hyperactivity in the other).

This sample's small size limits its utility (validity); however, the findings reinforce the clinical, albeit anecdotal, impression that OAD follows a chronic course. However, this disorder generally does not prevent the child from fulfilling at least basic academic and social demands. With especially stressful life events, however, exacerbations can be expected. If not treated, OAD may evolve into an adult generalized anxiety disorder or a social phobia.

Treatment

The reader is (once again) referred to Chapter 12, where the general principles and various treatment modalities for OAD are discussed. Specific treatment issues are addressed below.

Children with OAD have a strong motivation to perform well and to please others. This aspect of their personality in some ways facilitates treatment efforts; however, certain factors must be taken into account. When overanxiousness is a temperamental characteristic (such as in the "slow-to-warm-up" child), sufficient time and support must be given for the child to adapt at his or her own pace to a new environmental setting. A supportive and reassuring attitude from the therapist helps the child overcome feelings of insecurity or failure. Parental counseling and education aimed toward an improved understanding of the nature of their child's temperament is very effective in minimizing or removing environmental stresses. During crises precipitated by a frightening experience, it may become necessary to teach the child coping techniques. Desensitization methods may be used to help the child overcome a specific frightening situation or anxiety.

A family-oriented approach is indicated when chronically anxious parents, by virtue of their own insecurities and apprehensions, induce and prolong their child's anxieties.

Medication may be useful in certain situations. Anxiolytics, particularly minor tranquilizers such as diazepam, have proved effective in acute situations when used in conjunction with psychotherapy. Sedatives such as diphenhydramine hydrochloride may also be effective for the short-term management of acute anxiety with insomnia.

References

American Psychiatric Association: Diagnostic and Statistical Manual of Mental Disorders, 2nd Edition. Washington, DC, American Psychiatric Association, 1968

American Psychiatric Association: Diagnostic and Statistical Manual of Mental Disorders, 3rd Edition. Washington, DC, American Psychiatric Association, 1980

American Psychiatric Association: Diagnostic and Statistical Manual of Mental Disorders, 3rd Edition, Revised. Washington, DC, American Psychiatric Association, 1987

Bernstein GA, Garfinkel BD: School phobia: the overlap of affective and anxiety disorders. J Am Acad Child Psychiatry 25:235–241, 1986

Cantwell DP, Baker L: Psychiatric and behavioral characteristics of children with communication disorders. J Pediatr Psychol 5:161–178, 1980

Cantwell DP, Baker L: Psychiatric and learning disorders in children with speech and language disorders: a descriptive analysis. Advances in Learning and Behavioral Disabilities 4:29–47, 1985

Cantwell DP, Baker L: Stability and natural history of DSM-III childhood diagnoses. J Am Acad Child Adolesc Psychiatry 28(5):691–700, 1989

Hershberg SG, Carlson GA, Cantwell DP, et al: Anxiety and depressive disorders in psychiatrically disturbed children. J Clin Psychiatry 43:358–361, 1982

Jenkins R, Hewitt L: Types of personality structures encountered in child guidance clinics. Am J Orthopsychiatry 14:84–94, 1944

Last CG, Hersen M, Kazdin AE, et al: Comparison of DSM III separation anxiety and overanxious disorders: demographic characteristics and patterns of co-morbidity. J Am Acad Child Psychiatry 26:527–531, 1987

Chapter 9

Obsessive-Compulsive Disorder

*O*bsessions and compulsions of a minor nature are frequently encountered in young children. For example, the bedtime and feeding rituals of toddlers are often elaborate and persistent. Anxiety may be produced if these rituals are resisted by parents. In later childhood, "obsessional games" such as "step on a crack and break your mother's back" are often played. These are generally associated with obsessional fears recognized as unreasonable and absurd.

The earliest description of obsessive-compulsive disorder (OCD) in a child is given by Janet (1903), who reported a case of a 5-year-old boy with obsessive-compulsive symptoms. Freud's famous case, "rat man," first manifested his symptoms around 6 years of age. A number of other authors have since published case reports and their theories on the etiology of OCD. Hall (1935) described "obsessional states" in children that began as early as 4 years of age. Hall's report is considered by some to be the first modern account of OCD (Wolff and Rapoport 1988). Berman (1942), using retrospective chart analysis, diagnosed obsessive-compulsive neurosis in six children admitted to the children's ward at New York Bellevue Hospital.

A number of retrospective studies of adult obsessional patients also support the existence of this illness in children (Ingram 1961; Kringlen 1965; Lo 1967; Politt 1957; Warren 1960). Black (1974), reviewing these and other studies, concluded that in one-third of 357 adult cases the onset of OCD occurred between 5 and 15 years of age.

During the past 25 years a number of articles reporting specifically on OCD in children have been published (Hollingsworth et al. 1980; Judd 1965). All of these, however, are retrospective chart studies. The first effort to prospectively study this disorder was made by Adam (1973), who published a report on 49 children drawn from his clinical practice who were diagnosed with obsessive-compulsive neurosis. In 1977 National Institute of Mental Health researchers began a prospective study of this disorder using DSM-III (American Psychiatric Association 1980) criteria and a case-finding approach. Since this effort, they have published a number of reports discussing the epidemiology, phenomenology, and treatment of OCD (Flament et al. 1985; Rapoport et al. 1980; Wolff and Rapoport 1988).

OCD is not classified under childhood anxiety disorder in the DSM-III classification system. Unlike many other childhood psychiatric disorders, the clinical picture and phenomenology of OCD in children are identical to the clinical picture and phenomenology in adults; hence, adult diagnostic criteria may be applied without modification to children.

Some researchers question the inclusion of OCD under anxiety disorder (Behar et al. 1984; Berg et al. 1986; Rapoport et al. 1981); however, both old literature and current research have convincingly linked OCD and anxiety (Beech 1974; Carr 1974; Dollard and Miller 1950; Freud 1920; Jastrowitz 1878).

Epidemiology

Clinicians only infrequently encounter OCD in children, but according to some authorities underreporting likely exists (Jensen 1990). Berman (1942), in a 7-year retrospective review of 2,800 consecutive admissions to New York Bellevue Hospital's children's ward, diagnosed only six children (0.21%) with OCD. Judd (1965) reviewed 405 records of both inpatient and outpatient children at the University of California—Los Angeles (UCLA) and diagnosed only five cases (1.2%). Hollingsworth et al. (1980) reviewed 8,367 records of inpatients and outpatients at UCLA and found only 17 patients (0.2%) who met Judd's criteria for OCD.

However, a more accurate estimate of the incidence of OCD may be obtained by including adults with OCD who report onset of symptoms in early childhood. Politt (1957) reported childhood onset of OCD in 22% of adults diagnosed with OCD. Using a smaller sample, Warren (1960) reported a childhood onset of OCD in 60% of these adults, while Kringlen (1965) and Lo (1967) reported childhood onset in 20% and 36% of adults diagnosed with OCD, respectively.

Few researchers have studied OCD in the general population, rather than in a psychiatric population. Rutter et al. (1970) in the Isle of Wight Study surveyed more than 2,000 children aged 10–11 years and did not find a single case of OCD. Weissman et al. (1978) also failed to find any case of OCD among 511 members of a New Haven community. Rasmussen and Tsuang (1986), using a case-finding approach, advertised (including advertisements on television and in newspapers) but did not get a single response. Flament et al. (1985) developed a screening device for OCD and administered it to 5,000 students in a New Jersey school district, obtaining a prevalence rate of 0.33%. They felt that this underestimated the true rate due to the children's secretive attitude toward their illness and the possibility that severely disabled children were not participating. It is possible that similar factors may account for the low incidences uncovered in the Isle of Wight and other community surveys mentioned earlier. The possibility of underreporting is also supported by retrospective reports describing adults with OCD who had childhood onset of the condition but who did not seek any help until adulthood.

OCD may occur quite early in childhood. In Judd's (1965) series the average age of onset was 7.5 years, and in Hollingsworth et al.'s (1980) series it was 9.6 years with a range between 3 and 15 years. In the National Institute of Mental Health study (Rapoport et al. 1981) the mean age of onset reported was 9.5 years (SD = 4.1 years).

Earlier literature on OCD in children reported a slight preponderance of females (Anthony 1967). This finding, however, is not supported by more recent literature. In the study by Hollingsworth et al., 76% of the children with OCD were males. Similarly Rapoport (1986) reported a male-to-female ratio of 3:1, with males becoming ill an average of 2.5 years earlier. In Adam's (1973) series, boys outnumbered girls 4 to 1.

Clinical Picture

Most children and adolescents with OCD remain secretive about their illness for a long time, probably because of the "badness" or unacceptability of their thoughts (obsessions) and their embarrassment at the ritualistic behaviors (compulsions). These children perform their rituals secretly and generally escape the notice of even vigilant family members. Generally these children are compliant, conforming, and cooperative. They are described by their parents and teachers as "ideal children." Therefore, the notion that a serious problem may be brooding is frequently rejected. It is because of these factors that several years usually elapse between the onset of illness and beginning of treatment. The onset may be acute, in which case some precipitating event such as a psychological (Loeb 1986), physical (McKeon et al. 1984), or birth (Capstick and Seldrup 1977) trauma can be identified. In the majority of cases, however, the onset is insidious and the role of a precipitating event is generally unconvincing (Rapoport 1982).

Parents usually first become concerned about the child when ritualistic behaviors become frequent and disabling. Even at this stage most children persistently deny having any obsessive thoughts. Older children and adolescents are more willing to report their burdensome thoughts than are younger children. Symptoms of anxiety or depression, or both, are usually present. Anxiety symptoms become unbearable when the performance of rituals is hindered or blocked, either on the child's own initiative or by social circumstances. Depressive symptoms, primarily in response to the disabling nature of this condition, usually appear 1 or 2 years after the obsessive rituals begin (Rapoport 1982).

Three clinical subgroups of OCD are described in children and adolescents (Jensen 1990; Rapoport 1982, 1986). Patients in the first subgroup are isolated and withdrawn, with an anxious affect. They may be very suspicious, frequently to the extent of near-delusional thinking. These children are distinguished from schizophrenic children in that their associations are not truly loosened or disjointed. Similarly, they are differentiated from bipolar patients by the absence of hypomanic, tangential, or rambling associations. These children may have features of Asperger's syndrome with or without the avoidance of social interaction; they may also be mute with agitated depression.

The second group of children appear normal with affects ranging from anxiety to confusion to despair; such children have socialized normally with others but may show some minor conflicts with their family members. The third group of children with OCD are very likable, function in an exemplary manner in school, and may be outstanding athletes. Indeed, such children have been described as supernormal (Rapoport 1986). They are usually very concerned about their symptoms. Their anxiety and depression can be explained in terms of the thoughts and actions with which they are struggling.

Only a few children with OCD show an associated picture of Gilles de la Tourette's syndrome. However, a large number of patients with Tourette's syndrome are found to have associated obsessive-compulsive symptoms. Nee et al. (1980) reported on 50 consecutive cases of Tourette's syndrome; 34 of these patients also had OCD as defined by DSM-III.

Most children with OCD are usually of average intelligence, and the notion that OCD is a disease of the superintelligent is not supported by current research (Berg et al. 1982; Rapoport 1982).

Contamination, disorderliness, aggression, sexual acting-out, and failure to complete tasks are some of the obsessive themes of OCD children. The rituals are usually developed in order to eliminate or control the impact of these thoughts.

Family Psychopathology

Psychopathology among parents of OCD patients has been studied by a number of researchers (Adam 1977; Flament and Rapoport 1984; Hollingsworth et al. 1980; Kanner 1957; Kringlen 1965; Lewis 1935; Rasmussen and Tsuang 1984). Earlier studies documented a variety of psychopathologies, including but not limited to OCD, notably in parents (Hollingsworth et al. 1980) but also in siblings (Lewis 1935) and first-degree relatives (Rosenberg 1967). However, more recent studies (Flament and Rapoport 1984; Hoover and Insel 1984) do not support these earlier findings. Hoover and Insel (1984) systematically interviewed 174 family members of patients with OCD and found no OCD in any family members. Flament and Rapoport (1984), in the National Institute of Mental Health study, evaluated all first-degree relatives of 27 OCD children and adolescents. Family members older than 17 years were administered the Schedule for Affective Disorders and Schizophrenia—Life Time Version, minor siblings were given the Diagnostic Interview for Children and Adolescents, and diagnoses were based on DSM-III criteria. As in the study by Hoover and Insel, no parent had OCD and 61% had no lifetime diagnosis at all. Contradicting previous studies, no parents reported being meticulous or perfectionist (Kanner 1957), and there was no evidence of unusually strict child-rearing practices (Adam 1973; Kringlen 1965). The younger siblings, however, demonstrated a high frequency of impulse control disorder and learning disability. Nonetheless, no sibling had anxiety or OCD.

Diagnosis

A diagnosis of OCD is made when a patient has recurrent obsessions or compulsions that are sufficiently severe to cause marked distress and dysfunction (American Psychiatric Association 1987).

DSM-III-R Criteria for Diagnosis of OCD

A. Either obsessions or compulsions:
   Obsessions: 1, 2, 3, and 4:
   1. Recurrent and persistent ideas, thoughts, impulses, or images that are experienced, at least initially, as intrusive and senseless, e.g., a parent's having repeated impulses to kill a loved child, a religious person's having recurrent blasphemous thoughts.
   2. The person attempts to ignore or suppress such thoughts or impulses or to neutralize them with some other thought or action.
   3. The person recognizes that the obsessions are the product of his or her own mind, not imposed from without (as in thought insertion).
   4. If another Axis I disorder is present, the content of the obsession is unrelated to it; e.g., the ideas, thoughts, impulses, or images are not about food in the presence of an eating disorder, about drugs in the presence of a psychoactive substance use disorder, or guilty thoughts in the presence of a major depression.

   Compulsions: 1, 2, and 3
   1. Repetitive, purposeful, and intentional behaviors that are performed in response to an obsession, or according to certain rules or in a stereotyped fashion.
   2. The behavior is designed to neutralize or to prevent discomfort or some dreaded event or situation; however, either the activity is not connected in a realistic way with what it is designed to neutralize or prevent, or it is clearly excessive.
   3. The person recognizes that his or her behavior is excessive or unreasonable. (This may not be true for young children; it may no longer be true for people whose obsessions have evolved into overvalued ideas.)

B. The obsessions or compulsions cause marked distress, are time-consuming (take more than an hour a day), or significantly interfere with the person's normal routine, occupational functioning, or usual social activities or relationships with others.

A number of rating scales originally devised to assess OCD in adults have been modified for use in the adolescent population. The Maudsley Obsessive-Compulsive Questionnaire has 30 items falling into four general categories. These include "checking," "doubting and ruminating," "cleaning," and "obsessional slowing." Clark and Bolton (1985) used these instruments in adolescents and discovered that they only discriminated adolescents with OCD from normal adolescents in terms of total scores and checking factors.

Berg et al. (1986) have modified the Leyton Obsessive Inventory for Children (Leyton Obsession Inventory, Child Version [LOI-CV]) for use in adolescents. The LOI-CV was able to differentiate adolescents with OCD from normal controls. It was also found to be useful in measuring improvement among OCD patients during treatment with clomipramine.

The Diagnostic Interview Schedule for Children contains items that are instrumental for the diagnosis of OCD in children. Breslau (1987) assessed its efficacy for the diagnosis of OCD in children and concluded that the instrument overassesses obsessive-compulsive symptoms when administered by health care workers other than child psychiatrists. Questions tended to be misunderstood, and Breslau suggested that the Diagnostic Interview Schedule for Children be further modified, using longer, more-detailed questions that give specific examples that children could easily understand.

Differential Diagnosis

OCD should be distinguished from normal developmental rituals such as bedtime routines and obsessional games, which do not cause dysfunction or distress.

OCD should also be differentiated from Tourette's syndrome, in which preoccupation with coprolalia is coupled with a motor tic. However, Tourette's syndrome and OCD coexist in some people (American Psychiatric Association 1987).

Children with phobic anxiety may act in a phobic manner in the presence of, for example, dirt or contaminated material and may present a clinical picture resembling that of OCD. These children do not show an associated compulsion. Indeed, the distinction between OCD and phobic anxiety may be most difficult since in severe OCD, some phobic anxiety is always present (Rapoport 1982).

Other differential diagnoses of OCD include anorexia bulimia, schizoaffective disorder, major depressive disorder, Asperger's syndrome, autism, and separation anxiety disorder. Obsessional symptoms occasionally are present in schizophrenia, schizoaffective disorder, and major depression. The stereotypical behavior of schizophrenics is usually a manifestation of delusions rather then compulsions. Some OCD patients may develop an obsession that may in turn become an overvalued idea, hence resembling a delusion seen in schizophrenia. Unlike a patient with schizophrenia, however, a patient with OCD may be persuaded to "shake off" his overvalued belief.

In cases of depression, repetitive thoughts associated with guilt may be present and suggest OCD. In such instances accompanying vegetative symptoms such as eating and sleep disturbances, psychomotor retardation, anhedonia, and lack of energy will support the diagnosis of major depression.

Natural History

OCD in children frequently continues into adulthood. Freud (1920) has discussed the treatment (considered difficult) and prognosis (considered poor) of OCD. Few authors have reported success with psychoanalytic treatment (Bornstein 1949), family therapy (Fine 1973), or problem-solving therapy (O'Connor 1983), and the long-term success rate remains low.

Hollingsworth et al. (1980) followed 10 children with OCD during treatment at the UCLA Neuropsychiatric Institute. The treatment included for the most part outpatient psychotherapy (17.7 months, once or twice weekly). One patient also received behavior modification. Three patients were initially hospitalized. Seven of 10 patients continued to have OCD symptoms, although severity lessened following treatment. Long-term follow-up revealed continued difficulties with interpersonal relationships and a dislike for occupations in which obsessive-compulsive symptoms would surface. The long-term results in this sample were poor.

An improved outcome was reported by Apter et al. (1984), who combined psychotherapy with clomipramine and reported marked improvement in seven of eight adolescents with OCD. Four of these adolescents remained symptom free at follow-up 2–3 years later.

Elkins et al. (1980) reviewed outcome studies and concluded that 50% of children with OCD may not show appreciable improvement.

The factors influencing prognosis have been discussed by several authors (Baer and Minichiello 1986; Foa and Steketee 1977; Rachman and Hodgson 1980). A good premorbid adjustment and personality, mild symptoms, and short duration are associated with positive outcome. Noncompliance with treatment, a belief that the symptoms are necessary (i.e., bad consequences would occur if the rituals were not performed) (Foa and Steketee 1977), and the presence of a personality disorder were all associated with a poor prognosis (Baer and Minichiello 1986; Rachman and Hodgson 1980).

Etiology

A number of theories have been advanced to explain the etiology of OCD. These theories may be classified as psychoanalytic, neurological, and biochemical.

Psychoanalytic Theory

According to psychoanalytic theory, the child with OCD regresses from the oedipal to the anal-sadistic stage. The child uses isolation, displacement, reaction formation, and undoing as the defenses to counteract the anxiety produced by conflicts. According to this theory, it is these specific defenses that are responsible for the clinical picture of OCD. Earlier studies attributed the specific conflicts to harsh toilet training. However, more recent studies (Rapoport 1982) have failed to substantiate this relationship between toilet training and OCD.

Neurologic Theory

Gadelius, a Swedish physician, observed in 1896 that patients with OCD often demonstrated a number of neurological abnormalities such as mild tremors, rigid facies, akinesias, and hyperkinesis. On the basis of these findings he attributed OCD to a neurological lesion. More recently, neurological symptoms have been observed in some adolescents with sudden-onset OCD (Rapoport 1986). Interestingly, OCD has been produced experimentally in lab animals by stimulating the region of the cingulate gyrus.

OCD and Tourette's syndrome. In his original description, Tourette (1885) reported obsession in a woman with tics and vocalization. Many researchers have recently focused their efforts on studying OCD in patients with Tourette's syndrome. In one study (Pauls et al. 1986) 74% of patients with Tourette's syndrome had a significant number of obsessive-compulsive symptoms. The same authors also reported a significantly higher incidence of OCD among first-degree relatives of patients with Tourette's syndrome than in the general population. They concluded that the two diseases are etiologically related. Biederman et al. (1986) reported that 1.2% of the population carry a single major gene for Tourette's syndrome and that more than half express it in some form. Grad et al. (1987) reported that in their study 28% of the patients with Tourette's syndrome had OCD, compared with only 10% of the control group.

Twin studies. Lieberman (1984) studied 24 pairs of twins with OCD. A dizygotic pair was discordant for OCD. Of the 17 pairs of monozygotic twins, 12 pairs were concordant for OCD, while 5 were discordant.

Neurophysiologic studies. EEG abnormalities have been reported in 11–65% of OCD patients. Rapoport et al. (1981) found only one of nine (11%) children with OCD to have an abnormal EEG. Children with OCD also had abnormal sleep EEGs. All had short rapid-eye-movement latency, and 49% were left-handed (compared to a 10–20% incidence of left-handedness in the general population).

Grey-Walter (1966) produced OCD symptoms by stimulating the cingulate gyrus. Talairach et al. (1973) further localized the area to the anterior cingulate gyrus. Furthermore, psychosurgical lesions of the anterior cingulate gyrus have successfully treated the OCD symptoms (Kelly 1980).

By using brain imaging techniques, Behar et al. (1984) studied ventricle-to-brain ratios and found them to be significantly higher in adolescents with OCD than in controls. Baxter et al. (1987) studied the brain's glucose metabolic activity using positron-emission tomography. They found significantly greater metabolic activity in the orbital gyrus among OCD patients then among either depressed patients or normal controls. All OCD patients had abnormal activity in the dominant hemisphere. Significantly, those patients who responded to medication demonstrated increased metabolism in the caudate nucleus.

Biochemical Theory

OCD and neurotransmitters.   Serotonin, epinephrine, and dopamine have been implicated in the etiology of OCD. The serotonin hypothesis has received the most attention. According to this hypothesis, OCD is associated with impaired serotonin dysfunction. This hypothesis gained support from the clinical observation that patients with OCD improved with the use of clomipramine, a serotonin agonist (Stern and Wright 1980). Indeed, other serotonergic agonists such as L-tryptophan, lithium, and trazodone have also been efficacious. Flament et al. (1987) demonstrated that high pretreatment and low posttreatment platelet serotonin levels correlate highly with clinical improvement in OCD.

The norepinephrine theory is supported by the observation that clonidine, a specific noradrenergic agonist, improves the effectiveness of clomipramine in the treatment of OCD.

Dopaminergic pathways may also be involved in some cases of OCD. Both clomipramine and trimipramine have dopamine (D_2) receptor blockade properties, which may explain their effectiveness in the treatment of OCD.

However, it is likely that more than one neurotransmitter system is involved in the etiology of OCD.

Treatment

A number of other treatment modalities—including family therapy, behavior modification, psychoanalysis, and other psychotherapies—have been used in the treatment of OCD in children and adolescents with various success rates reported.

Psychotherapy

The effectiveness of psychoanalysis in the treatment of OCD is reported to be poor (Bornstein 1949; Loeb 1986). Some success has been

reported with dynamically oriented psychotherapy and supportive psychotherapy (Rapoport 1982). However, few research data are available
to objectively assess their efficacy in the treatment of OCD.

Family Therapy

Since the family often plays a role in the development of OCD, family
therapy is frequently recommended as an effective form of treatment
(Bolton et al. 1983; Fine 1973; Wolff and Rapoport 1988). Bolton et al.
(1983) and Hafner (1981) have discussed the goals and techniques of
family therapy in children and adolescents with OCD.

Behavior Therapy

Behavior therapy in adults with OCD is claimed to be successful,
especially exposure in vivo and response prevention techniques. The
literature on behavior therapy in children consists mainly of single case
reports (e.g., Zikis 1983). Other approaches include thought stopping
(Campbell 1973; Ownby 1983) and systemic desensitization (Phillips
and Wolpe 1981).

Psychopharmacotherapy

A number of drugs have been used for the treatment of OCD in
children. The use of antidepressants such as imipramine and
clomipramine has been based on the hypothesis that the neurotransmitters serotonin, epinephrine, and dopamine, either alone or in combination, are involved in the etiology of OCD. Clomipramine has been
found to be particularly effective in children and adolescents (Flament
et al. 1985; Rapoport et al. 1981; Warneke 1985).

References

Adam PL: Obsessive Children. New York, Penguin, 1973
Adam PL: Family characteristics of obsessive children. Am J Psychiatry
        128:1414–1417, 1977
American Psychiatric Association: Diagnostic and Statistical Manual of Mental
        Disorders, 3rd Edition. Washington, DC, American Psychiatric Association,
        1980

American Psychiatric Association: Diagnostic and Statistical Manual of Mental Disorders, 3rd Edition, Revised. Washington, DC, American Psychiatric Association, 1987

Anthony JE: Psychiatric disorders of childhood, II: psychoneurotic disorders, in Comprehensive Textbook of Psychiatry. Edited by Freedman M, Kafolan H. Baltimore, MD, Williams & Wilkins, 1967, pp 1387–1406

Apter A, Bernhout E, Tyano S: Severe obsessive compulsive disorder in adolescence. A report of eight cases. J Adolesc 7:349–358, 1984

Baer L, Minichiello WE: Behavior therapy for obsessive compulsive disorder, in Obsessive Compulsive Disorder. Edited by Jenike M, Baer L, Minichiello WE. Littleton, MA, PSG Publications, 1986, pp 45–75

Baxter CR, Phelps ME, Mazziota JC, et al: Local cerebral metabolic rates in obsessive compulsive disorder: a comparison with rates in unipolar depression and in normal controls. Arch Gen Psychiatry 44:211–218, 1987

Beech H: Obsessional States. London, Methuen, 1974

Behar D, Rapoport JL, Berg CJ, et al: Computerized tomography and neuropsychological test measures in adolescents with obsessive compulsive disorder. Am J Psychiatry 141:363–369, 1984

Berg C, Behar D, Cox C, et al: OCD in childhood. Paper presented at the annual meeting of the American Psychological Association, Washington, DC, May 1982

Berg LJ, Rappoport JL, Flament M: The Leyton Obsession Inventory—Child Version. J Am Acad Child Psychiatry 25:85–91, 1986

Berman L: The obsessive compulsive neurosis in children. J Nerv Ment Dis 95:26–39, 1942

Biederman J, Munir K, Knee D, et al: High rate of affective disorders in probands with attention deficit disorder and in their relatives: a controlled family study. Am J Psychiatry 144:330–333, 1986

Black A: The natural history of obsessional neurosis, in Obsessional States. Edited by Hoch PH, Zubin J. London, Methuen, 1974, pp 19–54

Bolton D, Collins S, Steinberg D: The treatment of obsessive compulsive disorder in adolescents: a report of fifteen cases. Br J Psychiatry 142:456–464, 1983

Bornstein L: The analysis of a phobic child. Psychoanal Study Child 3–4:181–226, 1949

Breslau N: Inquiring about the bizarre: false positive with DISC ascertainment of obsessions, compulsion and psychotic symptoms. J Am Acad Child Adolesc Psychiatry 26:639–644, 1987

Campbell LM: A variation of thought stopping in a 12-year-old boy: a case report. J Behav Ther Exp Psychiatry 4:69–70, 1973

Capstick N, Seldrup J: Obsessional states: a study in the relationship between abnormalities occurring at the time of birth and the subsequent development of obsessional symptoms. Acta Psychiatr Scand 56:427–431, 1977

Carr AT: Compulsive neurosis, a review of the literature. Psychol Bull 81:311–318, 1974

Clark DA, Bolton D: An investigation of two self report measures of obsessional phenomenon in obsessive compulsive adolescents (research note). J Child Psychol Psychiatry 26:429–437, 1985

Dollard J, Miller NE: Personality and Psychotherapy: An Analysis in Terms of Learning, Thinking and Culture. New York, McGraw-Hill, 1950

Elkins R, Rappoport J, Lipsky A: Obsessive compulsive disorder of childhood and adolescence. J Am Acad Child Psychiatry 19:511–524, 1980

Fine S: Family therapy and a behavioral approach to childhood obsessive compulsive neurosis. Arch Gen Psychiatry 28:695–697, 1973

Flament M, Rapoport JL: Childhood obsessive compulsive disorders, in New Findings in Obsessive Compulsive Disorder. Edited by Insel TR. Washington, DC, American Psychiatric Press, 1984, pp 24–43

Flament M, Rapoport JL, Murphy D, et al: Clomipramine treatment of childhood obsessive-compulsive disorder: a double-blind controlled trial. Arch Gen Psychiatry 42:977–983, 1985

Flament MF, Rapoport JL, Murphy DL, et al: Biochemical changes during clomipramine treatment of childhood obsessive compulsive disorder. Arch Gen Psychiatry 44:219–225, 1987

Foa EB, Steketee G: Emergent fears during treatment of three obsessive compulsives: symptom substitutions or deconditioning. J Behav Ther Exp Psychiatry 8:353–358, 1977

Freud S: Beyond the pleasure principle (1920), in The Standard Edition of the Complete Psychological Works of Sigmund Freud, Vol 18. Translated and edited by Strachey J. London, Hogarth Press, 1955, pp 7–64

Grad L, Pelcovitz D, Olsen M, et al: Obsessive compulsive symptomatology in children with Tourette's disorder. J Am Acad Child Adolesc Psychiatry 26:69–73, 1987

Grey-Walter W: Appendix A, in The Neurological Foundation of Psychiatry. Edited by Smythies R. Oxford, Blackwell, 1966

Hafner J: The treatment of obsessional neurosis in a family setting. Aust N Z J Psychiatry 15:145–157, 1981

Hall MB: Obsessive compulsive state in childhood. Arch Dis Childhood 10:49–59, 1935

Hollingsworth C, Tanguey P, Grossman L, et al: Long term outcome of obsessive compulsive disorder in children. J Am Acad Child Psychiatry 19:134–144, 1980

Hoover CF, Insel TR: Families of origin in obsessive compulsive disorder. J Nerv Ment Dis 172:207–215, 1984

Ingram IM: Obsessional illness in mental hospital patients. Journal of Mental Science 107:382–402, 1961

Janet P: Les Obsessions et la Psychiastreinie, Vol I. Paris, Felix Alean, 1903

Jastrowitz H: Discussion with Westphal. Archiv für Psychiatrie und Nerven-Krankheiten 8:750–755, 1878

Jensen JB: Obsessive compulsive disorder in children and adolescents, in Psychiatric Disorders in Children and Adolescents. Edited by Garfinkel B, Carlson G, Wheeler E. Philadelphia, PA, WB Saunders, 1990, pp 84–105

Judd L: Obsessive compulsive neurosis in children. Arch Gen Psychiatry 12:136–143, 1965

Kanner L: Child Psychiatry. Springfield, IL, Charles C Thomas, 1957

Kelly D: Anxiety and Emotion: Physiological Basis and Treatment. Springfield, IL, Charles C Thomas, 1980

Kringlen E: Obsessional neurotics: a long term follow up. Br J Psychiatry 111:709–722, 1965

Lewis A: Problems of obsessional illness. Proc R Soc Med 29:235–336, 1935

Lieberman J: Evidence for a biological hypothesis of obsessive compulsive disorder. Neuropsychobiology 11:14–21, 1984

Lo WH: A follow up study of obsessional neurotics in Hong Kong Chinese. Br J Psychiatry 113:823–832, 1967

Loeb LR: Traumatic contributions in the development of an obsessional neurosis in an adolescent. Adolesc Psychiatry 13:201–217, 1986

McKeon J, McCouffin P, Robinson P: Obsessive compulsive neurosis following head injury. A report of four cases. Br J Psychiatry 144:190–192, 1984

Nee LE, Caine ED, Polinsky RJ, et al: Gilles de la Tourette syndrome: clinical and family study of 50 cases. Ann Neurol 7:41–49, 1980

O'Connor JJ: Why can't I get hives? Brief strategic therapy with an obsessional child. Fam Process 22:201–209, 1983

Ownby RL: A cognitive behavioral intervention for compulsive handwashing with a thirteen-year-old boy. Psychology in the School 20:219–222, 1983

Pauls DL, Towbin KE, Leckman JF, et al: Gilles de la Tourette's syndrome and obsessive compulsive disorder: evidence supporting a genetic relationship. Arch Gen Psychiatry 43:1180–1182, 1986

Phillips D, Wolpe S: Multiple behavioral techniques in severe separation anxiety of a twelve-year-old. J Behav Ther Exp Psychiatry 12:329–332, 1981

Politt JD: The natural history of obsessional states, a study of 150 cases. Br Med J 1:194–198, 1957

Rachman SJ, Hodgson RJ: Obsessions and Compulsions. Englewood Cliffs, NJ, Prentice-Hall, 1980

Rapoport J: Childhood obsessive compulsive disorder, in Diagnosis and Treatment in Pediatric Psychiatry. Edited by Shaffer D, Erlhardt A, Greenhill L. New York, Macmillan, 1982

Rapoport JL: Annotation, childhood obsessive compulsive disorder. J Child Psychol Psychiatry 27:289–295, 1986

Rapoport J, Elkins R, Mikkelsen E: Clinical controlled trial of clomipramine in adolescents with obsessive compulsive disorder. Psychopharmacol Bull 16:61–63, 1980

Rapoport J, Elkins R, Langer DH, et al: Childhood obsessive compulsive disorder. Am J Psychiatry 138:1545–1554, 1981

Rasmussen S, Tsuang M: The epidemiology of obsessive compulsive disorder. J Clin Psychiatry 45:450–457, 1984

Rasmussen S, Tsuang M: Clinical characteristics and family history in DSM III obsessive compulsive disorder. Am J Psychiatry 143:317–322, 1986

Rosenberg C: Familial aspects of obsessional neurosis. Br J Psychiatry 113:405–413, 1967

Rutter M, Tizard J, Whitmore K: Education, Health and Behavior. London, Longman, 1970

Stern RS, Wright J: Clomipramine: plasma levels, side effects and outcome in obsessive compulsive neurosis. Postgrad Med J 56:134–139, 1980

Talairach J, Bancaud S, Geier S: The cingulate gyrus and human behavior. Electroencephalogr Clin Neurophysiol 34:45–51, 1973

Tourette G de la: Étude sur une affection nerveuse caraclerisee pa l'incoordination motrice, accompagne d'echolalic et de cospolalic. Arch Neurol 9:17–42, 158–200, 1885

Warneke LB: Intravenous chlorimipramine in the treatment of obsessional disorder: case report. J Clin Psychiatry 46:100–103, 1985

Warren W: Some relationship between the psychiatry of children and of adults. Journal of Mental Science 106:815–826, 1960

Weissman MM, Myers JK, Harding PS: Psychiatric disorders in U.S. urban community, 1975–1976. Am J Psychiatry 135:459–462, 1978

Wolff R, Rapoport J: Behavioral treatment of childhood obsessive compulsive disorder. Behav Modif 12:252–266, 1988

Zikis P: Treatments of an 11-year-old ritualizer and tiqueur girl with in vivo exposure and response prevention. Behavioral Psychology 11:75–81, 1983

Chapter 10

Phobic Disorders

*A*ny discussion of phobic disorders should begin with a clarification of three terms that are often used interchangeably but have distinct definitions: fear, phobia, and anxiety.

The term *fear* is derived from the old English word *faer,* which means "peril." Fear is a subjective unpleasant feeling that occurs in response to a recognizable source of danger, real or imagined. Fear is usually associated with a typical facial expression and a number of physiological changes such as an increase in the pulse and respiration rates, blood pressure, and muscle tension. The facial expression and physiological changes disappear as the source of danger is removed.

Anxiety is derived from the Latin word *anxius,* which means "troubled." Anxiety is a fear spread thin and is present without a recognizable specific source of danger. Anxious facies differs from the facial expression of fear and is generally persistent. The associated physiological symptoms depend on the intensity and duration of anxiety. Since the source of danger is unknown, the physiological concomitants of anxiety persist chronically.

The word *phobia* is derived from the ancient Greek word *phobos,* which means "dread." A phobia is an irrational fear that is intense and continues to persist in spite of the removal of the source of danger. The phobic reaction is not generally shared by other members of the same group, society, or culture.

Normal Fears in Children

Fears are common in children and are considered as a normal occurrence, peaking in prevalence at age 5 years and declining slowly thereafter (Jersild and Holmes 1935; MacFarlane et al. 1954). Fears can be grouped according to the age trends (Morris and Kratochwill 1983). In infancy, the most commonly encountered fears include the fears of strange objects and persons, noises, and falling. These fears reach their peak around age 2 years and disappear gradually thereafter. Fears of animals are rare in infancy but are frequently encountered around 3 years of age. Fear of the dark is most commonly reported by 4- to 5-year-old children. Some fears, such as fear of snakes and of meeting people, are not age dependent and may be reported at any age. The most common fears found in the 8- to 12-year-old age group are of political, home, and school-related situations (Croake and Knox 1973).

Historical Perspective

Since the phobias are usually tied in with the existence of real or imagined sources of danger, it is reasonable to presume that they have existed since antiquity and that ancient men and women have known and suffered from these conditions.

The earliest recorded case history of a phobic patient is attributed to Hippocrates (Frazier and Carr 1967). However, the current concept of agoraphobia owes its discovery to Westphal (1872), who published a monograph describing three male patients with fears of open or public places. His work played an important role in isolating the specific reaction that today is called *phobia.*

The present psychodynamic understanding of phobias is based on Freud's description of a 5-year-old boy, "little Hans," who was afraid to go out on the street because he was afraid that a horse might bite him (Freud 1909). Freud attributed this to Hans's competition with his father for the attention of his mother, resulting in hostile and aggressive feelings toward his father and consequent development of an intense fear of his father's retaliation. Freud explained that since such a hostile attitude toward one's father is unacceptable (ego dystonic), Hans displaced his fear and anxiety to a horse. According to Freud, in doing so Hans was able to avoid the object of his phobia and still could maintain a loving relationship with his father. Since Freud's formulation of a psychoanalytic theory of phobias, numerous other researchers (Arieti 1961; Deutsch 1932; Fenichel 1965; Lewin 1952; Ovesey 1962; Rado 1950) have contributed to the understanding of this condition.

Classification of Phobic Disorders

Phobias were first termed as anxiety hysteria. This choice of terminology reflected the psychoanalytic theory that dominated the thinking of the clinicians of that time. Subsequently, the terms "phobic neurosis" and "phobic reactions" were introduced.

In the DSM system of classification, phobias were first classified under the heading of psychoneurotic reactions (American Psychiatric Association 1952). This term was changed to phobic neurosis in DSM-II (American Psychiatric Association 1968) and was defined as an intense fear of an object or situation recognized as not dangerous and characterized by apprehension in the forms of faintness, fatigue, palpitation, perspiration, nausea, tremor, or panic. The DSM-I and DSM-II classifications of phobias were influenced by the psychoanalytic explanation of phobic reaction. In DSM-III (American Psychiatric Association 1980) the term "phobic neurosis" was changed to "phobic disorders." This change in the nomenclature represented a departure from the psychoanalytic thinking. In DSM-III specific criteria for the condition were identified, and the phobias were divided into three distinct subtypes: social phobia, agoraphobia, and simple phobia.

Epidemiology

Phobias are the most common forms of anxiety disorders. Between 5.1% and 12.5% of individuals of all ages and socioeconomic levels suffer from them in the United States (Robins et al. 1984). Whereas the prevalence of fears in children has been well studied, this has not been the case for the prevalence of clinical phobias in children. This is partly because phobias are relatively rare in children (Graziano et al. 1979; Miller et al. 1972). In the Isle of Wight study (Rutter et al. 1970), only 0.7% of children between the ages of 10 and 11 years were found to have clinically discernible phobias. Social phobias, such as fear of blushing, are the most common in adolescents and appear 2 years earlier in girls than in boys (Abe and Masui 1981).

Anderson et al. (1987) in a study of 11-year-old children from the general population in New Zealand found that 2.4% of the children had simple phobias and only 0.9% had social phobias. However, when the investigators used an additional information source as a requirement to make the diagnosis, none of the children were diagnosed to have simple or social phobias.

In another study (Strauss et al. 1988) of children and adolescents referred for the evaluation and treatment of anxiety disorders, 31%

were diagnosed with phobic disorders. Of these, 8.8% had social phobias; 10.5% had simple phobias; and 16.9% had a simple or social
phobia of school.

Sex differences are consistently reported in the prevalence of
phobias (Abe and Masui 1981; Anderson et al. 1987; Earls 1980), with
girls being overrepresented in the samples. Sex differences also exist
in the number and types of phobias reported. Girls report more fears
and are phobic of lightening, blushing, and going outdoors, while the
boys report a fear of talking in front of other people more often.

Clinical Picture

Essential Features

According to DSM-III-R (American Psychiatric Association 1987),
social phobia is a persistent fear of one or more situations in which the
person is exposed to possible scrutiny by others and fears that he or she
may do something or act in a way that will be humiliating or embarrassing. Speaking in public or choking on food when eating in front of
others are examples of social phobias.

In agoraphobia, there is a fear of being in places or situations from
which escape might be difficult or embarrassing. The individual often
fears that help might not be available if he or she develops a symptom
such as dizziness, cardiac distress, or loss of bladder or bowel control.
Because of these fears, the individual either stays home or needs a
companion when traveling.

According to DSM-III-R, the essential feature of simple phobia is
a persistent fear of and compelling desire to avoid an object or situation, as distinct from the fear of having a panic attack (as in panic
disorder) or of humiliation or embarrassment in a social situation (as in
social phobia). The exposure to the phobic object or situation invariably provokes an immediate anxiety response, and the person recognizes the irrationality and excessiveness of his or her anxiety. Some
common examples of simple phobias found in children and adolescents include the fear of animals, heights, darkness, and thunderstorms
(Ollendick 1979).

Associated Features

Children with social phobias report depression more often than do children with simple phobias (Strauss et al. 1988). Depression is also found as a concurrent diagnosis in one-third of children with school phobia (Last et al. 1987). Multiple mild fears are also commonly reported in association with school phobia. Among the anxiety disorder diagnoses, overanxious disorder is found to be commonly associated with phobic disorders. In a clinic sample of phobic children, Strauss et al. (1988) found that 38% of children with school phobia, 50% of children with simple phobia, and 67% of children with social phobia had a concurrent diagnosis of overanxious disorder.

Differential Diagnosis

Social phobias should be distinguished from shyness and from normal fears of embarrassment commonly seen in this age group. In the latter cases the anxiety is not as excessive and does not produce dysfunction. Social phobia should also be distinguished from overanxious disorder. In overanxious disorder the anxiety is generalized and nonspecific to a situation, and avoidance of the situation is not present. Other associated symptoms of overanxious disorder, such as a generalized feeling of tension, somatic complaints, and anxious facies, are not present in phobic children.

The distinction between social phobias and avoidant disorder is made on the basis of the history. The child with avoidant disorder avoids all social situations involving unfamiliar persons. Other psychiatric conditions such as major depression, schizophrenia, and obsessive-compulsive disorder may have anxiety and avoidance of social situations as associated symptoms and should not be confused with social phobias.

Social phobia should also be separated from simple phobia, in which case the anxiety and avoidance involve a specific circumscribed object, person, animal, etc. A child or adolescent with posttraumatic stress disorder may avoid a situation or object associated with actual trauma, e.g., a closet or a swimming pool. A number of normal and psychiatric conditions may mimic the clinical picture of simple phobia. In normal fear, an age trend can be readily recognized, and the associated anxiety is not excessive. In schizophrenic adolescents, avoidant behavior may be observed sometimes as part of delusional thinking. A careful mental status examination usually reveals that the affected individual does not view his or her anxiety as excessive. In patients with obsessive-compulsive disorder who avoid certain objects, the associated anxiety is usually reduced by compulsive acts.

Natural History

The current understanding regarding the outcome of phobic disorders is derived from retrospective studies of adults. Most studies identify the age of onset of the phobic disorder as an important factor underlying the stability of the condition. The phobias that have their onset in adolescence (e.g., agoraphobia) are more persistent than the ones that start early (e.g., simple phobia). In a study by Sheehan et al. (1981), 31% of the adults with simple phobia reported that their phobia began before age 9 years, and 26% reported it began between 10 and 19 years. In another study (Agras et al. 1972), 100% of the phobias observed in children and adolescents were remitted within 5 years.

Agoraphobia runs a more chronic course in adults and usually has its onset in adolescence (Sheehan et al. 1981).

Treatment

The treatment of phobias in children is not well studied, and the literature on the subject is limited mostly to single case reports. Three intervention approaches are often employed: modeling, cognitive-behavioral technique, and systematic desensitization.

Modeling

With this technique, the phobic child is first shown a videotaped or live model approaching the feared object and is then encouraged to do the same. Modeling is found to be an effective treatment modality for childhood simple phobias (Harris 1983) if it is used in association with gradual exposure and live models (Graziano et al. 1979).

The efficacy of the modeling technique for the treatment of social phobias is questioned by some authors (Graziano et al. 1979). However, O'Connor (1969) has reported good results with this technique in socially withdrawn and fearful children.

Cognitive-Behavioral Technique

This technique involves helping the child to use self-statements that reflect coping and competency (for example, "I am a brave boy or girl") or fear-reduction statements (for example, "swimming is a fun sport"). Cognitive and behavioral approaches are found to be effective in reducing anxiety and avoidance in phobic children (Kanfer et al. 1975). However, the effectiveness of this technique as a treatment for phobic children requires further study (Harris 1983).

Systematic Desensitization

The effectiveness of the desensitization technique alone for the treatment of childhood phobias is limited (Kelley 1976; Miller et al. 1972). However, when used in association with modeling and contingency management approaches, systemic desensitization was found to produce positive results (Lietenberg and Callahan 1973; Mann and Rosenthal 1969).

References

Abe K, Masui T: Age-sex trends of phobic and anxiety symptoms in adolescents. Br J Psychiatry 138:297–302, 1981

Agras WS, Chapin HH, Oliveau DC: The natural history of phobia. Arch Gen Psychiatry 26:315–317, 1972

American Psychiatric Association: Diagnostic and Statistical Manual: Mental Disorders. Washington, DC, American Psychiatric Association, 1952

American Psychiatric Association: Diagnostic and Statistical Manual of Mental Disorders, 2nd Edition. Washington, DC, American Psychiatric Association, 1968

American Psychiatric Association: Diagnostic and Statistical Manual of Mental Disorders, 3rd Edition. Washington, DC, American Psychiatric Association, 1980

American Psychiatric Association: Diagnostic and Statistical Manual of Mental Disorders, 3rd Edition, Revised. Washington, DC, American Psychiatric Association, 1987

Anderson JC, Williams S, McGee R, et al: DSM-III disorders in pre-adolescent children. Arch Gen Psychiatry 44:69–76, 1987

Arieti SA: A re-examination of the phobic symptom and of symbolism in psychopathology. Am J Psychiatry 118:106, 1961

Croake JW, Knox FH: The changing nature of children's fears. Child Study Journal 3:91–105, 1973

Deutsch H: Psycho-analysis of the Neuroses. London, Hogarth Press, 1932

Earls F: Prevalence of behavior problems in three-year-old children: a cross national replication. Arch Gen Psychiatry 37:1153–1157, 1980

Fenichel O: The Psychoanalytic Theory of Neurosis. New York, WW Norton, 1965

Frazier SH, Carr AC: Phobic reaction, in Comprehensive Textbook of Psychiatry. Edited by Freedman AM, Kaplan HI. Baltimore, MD, Williams & Wilkins, 1967, pp 899–911

Freud S: Analysis of a phobia in a five-year-old boy (1909), in The Standard Edition of the Complete Psychological Works of Sigmund Freud, Vol 10. Translated and edited by Strachey J. London, Hogarth Press, 1955, pp 5–149

Graziano A, DeGiovanni IS, Garcia K: Behavioral treatment of children's fears: a review. Psychol Bull 86:804–830, 1979

Harris SL: Behavior therapy with children, in The Clinical Psychology Handbook. Edited by Hersen M, Kazdin AE, Bellack AS. Elmsford, NY, Pergamon, 1983

Jersild AT, Holmes FB: Methods of overcoming children's fears. J Psychol 1:75–104, 1935

Kanfer F, Karoly P, Newman A: Reduction of children's fear of the dark by competence-related and situational threat-related verbal cries. J Consult Clin Psychol 43:251–258, 1975

Kelley CK: Play desensitization of fear of darkness in preschool children. Behav Res Ther 14:79–81, 1976

Last C, Francis G, Hersen M, et al: Separating anxiety and school phobia: a comparison using DSM III criteria. Am J Psychiatry 144:653–657, 1987

Lewin BD: Phobic symptoms and dream interpretation. Psychoanal Q 21:295, 1952

Lietenberg H, Callahan E: Reinforced practice and reduction of different kinds of fears in adults and children. Behav Res Ther 11:19–30, 1973

MacFarlane JW, Allen L, Honzik MP: A Developmental Study of the Behavior Problems of Normal Children Between Twenty-one Months and Fourteen Years. Berkeley, CA, University of California Press, 1954

Mann J, Rosenthal TL: Vicarious and direct counter conditioning of test anxiety through individual and group desensitization. Behav Res Ther 7:359–367, 1969

Miller LC, Barrett CL, Hampe E, et al: Comparison of reciprocal inhibition, psychotherapy and waiting list control for phobic children. J Abnorm Psychol 79:269–279, 1972

Morris RJ, Kratochwill TR: Treating Children's Fears and Phobias: A Behavioral Approach. Elmsford, NY, Pergamon, 1983

O'Connor RD: Modification of social withdrawal through symbolic modeling. J Applied Behav Anal 2:15–22, 1969

Ollendick TH: Fear reduction techniques with children, in Progress in Behavior Modification, Vol 8. Edited by Hersen M, Eisler R, Miller P. New York, Academic, 1979

Ovesey L: Fear of vocational success: a phobic extension of the paranoid reaction. Arch Gen Psychiatry 7:82, 1962

Rado S: Emergency behavior with an introduction to the dynamics of conscience, in Anxiety. Edited by Hoch P, Zubin J. New York, Grune & Stratton, 1950, p 150

Robins LN, Helzer JE, Weissman MM, et al: Life time prevalence of specific psychiatric disorders in three sites. Arch Gen Psychiatry 41:949–958, 1984

Rutter M, Tizard J, Whitmore S: Education, Health and Behavior. London, Longman, 1970

Sheehan DV, Sheehan KE, Minichiello WE: Age of onset of phobic disorders: a re-evaluation. Compr Psychiatry 22:544–553, 1981

Strauss GC, Lease CL, Last CG, et al: Overanxious disorder: an examination of development differences. J Abnorm Child Psychol 16:433–443, 1988

Westphal C: Die Agoraphobic: Eine neuropathische Ercheiming. Arch Psychiatry Nervenky 3:138, 1872

Chapter 11

Panic Disorder

Conventional clinical wisdom has been that panic disorder is found only among adults. However, evidence derived from several studies suggest that this symptom pattern does occur before puberty (Van Winter and Strickler 1984; Vitiello et al. 1987).

Retrospectively taken childhood histories of adults with panic disorder, studies of the parents of children with anxiety disorders, and studies of children with depressed and anxious parents support the association between adult and childhood anxiety disorders. More specifically, studies of adults with panic disorder have revealed cases of onset of panic disorder in childhood (Sheehan et al. 1981).

Moreau et al. (1989) presented diagnostic data on seven children, aged 11 to 23 years, who were found to have panic symptoms: shortness of breath, palpitations, chest pain, choking, dizziness, sweating, trembling, tingling, fears of death, and hot/cold flashes. These symptoms were similar to those found in adults with panic disorder. Feelings of panic, anxiety, or fear occurred suddenly and were accompanied by multiple physical and psychological symptoms. All of the children had other diagnoses, most commonly major depression and separation anxiety disorder (SAD). The onset of panic disorder either occurred in conjunction with SAD or major depression or followed the onset of SAD by at least several months.

Hence, these findings suggest that panic disorder can occur before puberty. The symptom pattern and comorbidity with depression are similar to those found in adults. Furthermore, these findings, if replicated, would underscore the importance of including a systematic assessment of panic disorder as part of a general psychiatric workup for children.

Similar results confirming that panic attacks are not confined to adults were reported by Hayward et al. (1989). In this study, the authors interviewed a sample of ninth graders to determine the prevalence of panic attacks in young adolescents. They reported a lifetime prevalence of 11.6% for interview-determined panic attacks in 95 ninth graders. Obviously, the observed frequency of panic attacks varies according to the method of assessment, number of symptoms required for the diagnosis, time period considered, and population studied. Results of this study also show considerable comorbidity with anxiety and depression in the ninth graders, as well as an association between panic attacks and cigarette smoking.

The continuity of childhood panic disorder into adulthood, as well as the clinical course and actual prevalence of panic disorder, is unknown. Also, while there is strong evidence for the utility of pharmacological and behavioral treatments of panic in adults (American Psychiatric Press 1988), the efficacy of these treatments in children is unknown.

References

American Psychiatric Press Review of Psychiatry, Vol 7. Edited by Frances AJ, Hales RE. Washington, DC, American Psychiatric Press, 1988

Hayward C, Killen JD, Taylor CB: Panic attacks in young adolescents. Am J Psychiatry 146:1061–1062, 1989

Moreau DL, Weissman M, Warner V: Panic disorder in children at high risk for depression. Am J Psychiatry 146:1059–1060, 1989

Sheehan DV, Sheehan KE, Minichiello WE: Age of onset of phobic disorders: a reevaluation. Compr Psychiatry 22:544–553, 1981

Van Winter JT, Strickler GB: Panic attack syndrome. J Pediatr 105:661–665, 1984

Vitiello B, Behar D, Wolfson S, et al: Panic disorder in prepubertal children (letter). Am J Psychiatry 144:525–526, 1987

Chapter 12

Posttraumatic Stress Disorder

*T*he clinical picture of posttraumatic stress disorder (PTSD), an anxiety disorder classified in DSM-III-R (American Psychiatric Association 1987), includes the following criteria:

1. The person has experienced an event that is outside the range of usual human existence and that would be markedly distressing to almost anyone.
2. The traumatic event is persistently reexperienced.
3. There is continued avoidance of stimuli associated with the trauma or numbing of general responsiveness.
4. Symptoms of increased arousal persist that were not present before the trauma.

This anxiety disorder can occur at any age, and increased attention has been focused on the symptoms of PTSD in children who have experienced extreme stress.

The first criterion listed above emphasizes the unusual and extreme nature of the stressor. Two stressors most likely to induce posttraumatic stress symptoms are 1) serious threat to the child's family members or a close friend's life and 2) witnessing injury or death as a result of an accident or physical violence. Specific experiences—such as witnessing the grotesque or hearing cries of distress—intensify the recall of the traumatic experience. The greater the impact, the more likely there will be a traumatic response. Furthermore, children appear to respond more severely and their actions last longer when the traumatic event is associated with human accountability (e.g., human error), in contrast to a natural disaster.

Not all children are equally at risk of developing PTSD. At highest risk are those who were in immediate threat of death, who were present in the impact zone, who suffered severe injury, and who witnessed the death or injury of family members or friends.

There are no estimates of the percentage of children who have experienced PTSD symptoms. However, data pertaining to disasters and domestic violence suggest the potential extent of children's exposures to stressors. For example, in 1985 there were 19,000 homicides in the United States, and between 10% and 20% of all homicides are witnessed by children (Pynoos 1990).

Reexperiencing phenomena demonstrates how elements of the traumatic experience remain active in children's mental life. Children often experience intrusive recollections in the form of recurrent thoughts, images, or sounds; traumatic dreams; repetitive and unrewarding play; reenactment behavior of some part of the traumatic experience; distress at traumatic reminders (e.g., after a tornado, children may become anxious any time it is windy); avoidance of thoughts, feelings, locations, or situations associated with the trauma; reduced interest in usual activities; feelings of being alone or detached; restricted emotional range; memory distortions; loss of acquired skills; and change in orientation toward the future.

DSM-III-R establishes a separate criterion for the somatic symptoms of arousal, highlighting the physiological as well as psychological substrate of PTSD. Such reactions include sleep disturbance, irritability, difficulty concentrating, and hypervigilance.

In addition to the general symptom profile noted above, each age group seems vulnerable to certain behavioral changes. For example, preschool children are most likely to exhibit decreased verbalization and cognitive confusion. School-age children are more apt to react to trauma with aggressive or inhibited behavior. Finally, adolescents often show a premature movement toward independence or an increased dependence.

The clinical course of PTSD in children and adolescents is variable, depending on the severity, duration, and personal impact of the experience. DSM-III-R requires a duration of at least 1 month before the diagnosis is warranted to permit early detection of the disorder and to exclude persons with only a transient stress reaction.

Successful intervention requires triaging and screening for children at risk and reducing stress-induced disturbances in children undergoing normative reactions. Strategies focus on strengthening individual and family coping capacities, as well as decreasing adverse influences on recovery. Because PTSD is a new classification, the diagnosis should be approached conservatively until more research has been done.

References

American Psychiatric Association: Diagnostic and Statistical Manual of Mental Disorders, 3rd Edition, Revised. Washington, DC, American Psychiatric Association, 1987

Pynoos RS: Posttraumatic stress disorder in children and adolescents, in Psychiatric Disorders in Children and Adolescents. Edited by Garfinkel BD, Carlson GA, Weller EB. Philadelphia, PA, WB Saunders, 1990, pp 48–63

Chapter 13

Developmental Perspectives

*D*evelopmental psychology is concerned with the processes and mechanisms of development from infancy through adulthood, with an interest in the discontinuities as well as the continuities. The adjective "developmental" implies that experiences or processes during a given phase of life may modify an individual's set of responses at a later point (Rutter 1986). From a developmental-psychopathology perspective, inquiry is directed toward the links (or lack thereof) between normal behavioral emotions and clinical disorders, as well as the parallels (or lack thereof) between the "normal" and "abnormal" adaptive responses to stress.

Although the developmental aspects of childhood psychiatric disorders represent a relatively new field of interest, a number of investigators (e.g., Achenbach 1982; Garber 1984) have concluded that effective diagnosis of childhood disorders requires a significant knowledge of child development. By addressing such issues as the continuities and discontinuities between child and adult psychopathology, contributions can be made toward the more accurate diagnosis of childhood disorders.

Eisenberg (1977) argued that the developmental viewpoint represents an essential unifying concept in the psychiatry of both adults and children. Development encompasses not only the roots of behavior (prior to physical maturation and in physical influences) but also the modulations of that behavior by present circumstances. Developmentalists are pursuing and must continue to pursue questions such as the following: Does age influence a child's ability to experience or express anxious feelings? Does the manner of expression alter with development? Is the expression of anxious feelings at one age dependent upon prior maturational changes or experiences at an earlier point in time? Each of these questions is fundamental to a developmental approach (Rutter 1986).

Children are continually growing and maturing organisms, both quantitatively and qualitatively; they are not "miniature adults." At different ages and stages they have unique life experiences and may not manifest symptomatology in the same way as adults. It is natural, then, to question whether or not adult diagnostic criteria are applicable to diagnosis in children. The erroneous assumption that adult-based categories accurately reflect disorders in childhood (without independent validation) has been termed "adultomorphism" (Phillips et al. 1975). In opposition to this diagnostic method, Gelfand and Peterson (1985) have argued that there is no guarantee that child and adult forms of a disturbance will be manifested in the same fashion. Furthermore, proponents of adultomorphic classification systems fail to recognize that pathology is usually age-dependent (Peterson et al. 1988).

Thus, a major obstacle to progress in developmental-psychopathology research has been the lack of a reliable classification system for emotional and behavioral problems in children (Garber 1984). Currently, there is no universally accepted classification scheme for childhood psychopathology—instead, several systems have emerged, including DSM-III and DSM-III-R (American Psychiatric Association 1980, 1987) and the scheme developed by the Group for the Advancement of Psychiatry (1966). Skepticism about these schemes stems from an increasing awareness that children indeed develop more rapidly than do adults. Consequently, the extent to which measurement at any one point in time adequately portrays their "average" or "typical" functioning is limited. Hence, the difficulties a child may encounter and the ways in which these difficulties are responded to can vary across relatively brief time spans. However, developmental psychopathology does offer new conceptualizations and insights into dysfunctional behavior of children, and below we attempt to further this knowledge.

Developmental Issues in Relation to Childhood Anxiety

Distinctions have often been made between fear, which is focused on a specific object or situation, and anxiety, which is nonspecific and diffuse in nature (e.g., Miller et al. 1974). However, DSM-III recognizes that both fear and anxiety have similar cognitive, affective, and physiological patterns, which include, for example, thoughts of imminent danger. The developmental literature tends to focus on specific fears with the implication that fear and anxiety can be used interchangeably (Campbell 1986).

First, it is important to note that many individual differences exist in the expression of fear during childhood, and these are influenced by such factors as temperamental characteristics, the specific situational context, age, developmental stage, and so forth. Hence, empirical investigations of children's fears are rendered more difficult since behavioral responses are such a poor indicator of fear (Campbell 1986).

Development of Fears

The development of fears has been discussed within a variety of frameworks. The ethological perspective maintains that the human organism is genetically programmed to fear certain types of situations and stimuli, such as loud noises and darkness (Bowlby 1973). In an evolutionary sense, these innate fears are both natural and adaptive in that they serve to protect people from harmful situations. Along these lines, preprogrammed infant behaviors such as crying and clinging are assumed to promote and maintain proximity to an attachment figure, ensuring protection from harmful exposures (Campbell 1986).

Other fears have been explained from a cognitive-developmental viewpoint. Fear of strangers seems to require some dependence on previous experiences in the world. These learned fears may be based on recall of unpleasant experiences involving familiar objects or situations, such as mother-child separation (Lewis and Rosenblum 1974). Still other learned fears may be responses to novel or unfamiliar situations.

As children's cognitive abilities develop to permit language, their fears change. In the early preschool years, children are able to anticipate harmful or frightening events; hence, fears of animals, the dark, and imaginary creatures begin to emerge (Graziano et al. 1979). In contrast, younger school-age children fear frightening dreams, ghosts, and monsters—fears that also diminish with age. Realistic fears, however, while infrequent in young children, become more common by early adolescence (Bauer 1976). Results of an interview with kindergarten, second, and sixth graders revealed that kindergartners and second graders were more likely to report fears of monsters, ghosts, etc., whereas sixth graders were more concerned about bodily injury and physical danger. Hence, Bauer (1976) concludes that specific fears are associated with each developmental stage. Early on, fears reflect the formless and imaginary. With children's greater experience and increased control over their environment, their fears become more realistic. Fears of bodily injury as well as concern about social interactions tend to increase with age from the middle school years into adolescence.

The stability of fourth graders' fears was explored in a study by Emde and Schmidt (1978). A follow-up assessment 1 year later revealed that both the number and types of reported fears remained remarkably stable. Fears of bodily harm, animals, and disaster were most frequently noted. It has been found, though, that particular types of fears appear to develop in middle to late childhood and remain persistent throughout life. Examples of these types of fears include fear of loss, bodily injury, and social anxiety. Thus, while fear of monsters and the dark may decrease as a function of cognitive and social development, realistic fears developing in adolescence may persist longer (Campbell 1986). Interestingly, age at onset of a phobia is apparently related to the phobia's stability over time. Agras et al. (1972) found that phobias in young persons were far less persistent than phobias in adults over 20 years of age. In fact, all of the untreated phobias in children and adolescents disappeared within 5 years. Agras and colleagues also noted that more specific and focused fears were associated with better long-term outcome.

Development and Various Anxiety Disorders

The term "separation anxiety" refers to the protest when the caregiver departs and the distress and anxiety caused by his or her absence (e.g., Weinraub and Lewis 1977). The determinants of separation anxiety are complex and many: the quality of the mother-infant attachment (Ainsworth et al. 1978), the age of the child (Stayton et al. 1973), and the nature of the situation (Weinraub and Lewis 1977) are just a few of the variables that affect the intensity of the child's reaction.

Based on a review of the literature, children with separation anxiety disorder are usually younger than children with other anxiety subtypes. For example, Last et al. (1987c) found that children with separation anxiety were usually prepubertal, whereas children with school phobia tended to be postpubertal. Likewise, in a study investigating comorbidity among childhood anxiety disorders, Last et al. (1987a) presented the mean age of children with various anxiety disorders. Children with separation anxiety disorder ($n = 24$) had a mean age of 8.9 years, whereas those with overanxious disorder ($n = 11$) and phobia ($n = 11$) had mean ages of 10.8 and 14.2 years, respectively.

In another study by Last et al. (1987b), separation anxiety and overanxious disorders were compared along a variety of dimensions, including age. Almost all children with separation anxiety ($n = 22$) were prepubertal (91%), while overanxious children ($n = 26$) were generally postpubertal (69%). Also, children with both overanxious disorder and separation anxiety were older than children with only separation anxiety but younger than children with only overanxious disorder. The authors correctly note that this pattern raises the possibility that separation anxiety may in fact be a risk factor for the later development of overanxious disorder. In other words, the presence of one anxiety disorder may predispose the person to develop a second anxiety disorder.

Although lab studies investigating separation anxiety have the inherent confounding factors of reactions to unfamiliar people behaving in unfamiliar manners, these studies have revealed some consistent findings. Most 1- to 2-year-olds do become distressed when left alone or with a stranger in a strange environment (Ainsworth et al. 1978; Weinraub and Lewis 1977). According to the ethological perspective described earlier, the absence of mother in a strange environment may be interpreted by the child as a sign of danger. However, when the infant initiates separation in order to explore other rooms and the mother is nearby, separation does not result in distress (Rheingold and Eckerman 1970).

For the most part, separation anxiety has an acute onset that often occurs after a major stressor, such as moving to a new school or beginning preschool (e.g., McGrew 1972). Slightly older children have less separation anxiety distress on the first day of preschool, however, if they have had previous peer group experiences (Feldbaum et al. 1980). Separation anxiety has also been noted to occur following prolonged vacations from school or absence (e.g., due to illness) (Last 1987). Additionally, during certain developmental transitions—such as moving from elementary to junior high school—the incidence of the disorder increases. It is common for a child who presents with the disorder at 10, 11, or 12 years of age to have a history of separation anxiety during kindergarten or first grade. This reveals the continuous nature of anxiety, as well as the changes in clinical manifestations of anxiety, which vary for each age group.

While studies investigating the effects of maternal employment and day care on the child's well-being have generally found that this mother-child separation has not had major negative effects on the child (e.g., Hoffman 1979), there are indications that divorce has profound effects on children (e.g., Wallerstein and Kelly 1980). During this tumultuous time, children—ranging from toddlers to adolescents—often experience profound sadness, anger, guilt, and concern about current nurturance and future living arrangements; these feelings may be manifested in a variety of symptoms, such as separation distress.

In contrast to separation anxiety disorder, overanxious disorder appears to be more chronic. This condition is characterized by pervasive anxiety that is not focused on a specific object or situation. Children diagnosed with this disorder are usually overconcerned with evaluation from others, are constantly needing reassurance from others, are excessively worried about future and past events, and are generally self-conscious. It is typical for children who present at a mental health setting to have a several-year history of the disorder without remission (Last 1987). Although the disorder does not remit spontaneously, it may become more intense during intense stress or developmental transitions. Furthermore, preliminary evidence suggests that overanxious disorder during childhood or adolescence may lead to the individual's developing generalized anxiety disorder as an adult (Last et al. 1987b).

A study by Strauss et al. (1988b) described the manifestation of overanxious disorder in 55 children (aged 5–11 years) compared with adolescents (aged 12–19 years). More specifically, the two age groups were compared by evaluating prevalence, sociodemographic characteristics, symptom expression, association with other forms of maladjustment, and self-reported anxiety and depression. Both differences and similarities between the two groups emerged. Sixty-six percent of the older children met most of the diagnostic criteria for overanxious disorder, compared with only 35% of the younger children. Also, the older children more frequently had a concurrent diagnosis of major depression or simple phobia, whereas the younger children more commonly exhibited concurrent separation anxiety disorder or attention-deficit disorder. Older children were also more likely to report high levels of anxiety and depression on various self-report measures. Strauss and colleagues proposed several different interpretations for the finding that the older children exhibited more overanxious symptoms than did the younger children. The authors felt it could be due to developmental differences in cognitive abilities or simply to a longer duration of symptoms in the older group.

The groups were similar in that prevalence of overanxious diagnosis and socioeconomic variables did not differ between the age groups in this sample. Furthermore, the frequency of specific overanxious symptoms did not appear to change with age.

Although it was not surprising that the younger group had concurrent separation anxiety disorder more frequently than did the older group, the high comorbidity of overanxious disorder and attention-deficit disorder in the younger group was quite noteworthy. Strauss et al. argue that this may support the general finding that the severity and number of attention-deficit symptoms decline in children with increasing age (e.g., Barkley 1981). Finally, the high degree of concurrent anxiety and affective disorders in both groups of children raises the question of the purity of overanxious disorder and the need for greater distinction among anxiety disorder subtypes.

In another investigation by Strauss et al. (1988a), which focused on the association between anxiety and depression, results showed that older children (aged 12–17 years) with an anxiety disorder had a significantly higher number of concurrent diagnoses of depression than did younger children (aged 5–11 years) with an anxiety disorder. This pattern of results suggests that the extent of overlap between anxiety and depression may be a function of the age of the anxious population. A temporal sequence hypothesis has even been formulated to explain such age differences (Stavrakaki et al. 1987); since anxiety (without depression) is more common in younger age groups, then it is possible that anxious children may become depressed adults.

A developmental perspective of psychopathology among a community sample of children and adolescents was provided by Kashani et al. (1989). This study attempted to integrate epidemiological methods, current diagnostic classifications, and developmental psychopathology in order to provide data on normal and abnormal changes over time. The two independent variables included in the study were gender and age. The differences were examined on dependent variables such as frequency of diagnoses, diagnostic symptom levels, and levels of functioning in various spheres. In addition, parental reports were compared with child reports for all analyses.

The subjects in this study were 210 children and adolescents; there were 70 students from each of three age groups (8-, 12-, and 17-year-olds), half girls and half boys. Psychopathology in the child was measured with the Child Assessment Schedule (CAS) (Hodges et al. 1982) and the P-CAS (administered to the parent).

Anxiety was the most frequently reported symptom in all three age groups, irrespective of informant. More specific results revealed that anxiety symptoms such as separation concerns decreased with age, whereas specific fears and social embarrassment increased with age. This suggests that while overall rates of anxiety remain stable throughout developmental transitions, the focus of the anxiety changes; during early development, concerns are more amorphous and family oriented, but as the child ages, interpersonal and peer concerns dominate. Interestingly, while both males and females showed similar trends with regard to anxiety, only females became more anxious over time about competence.

A later developmental study by Kashani and Orvaschel (1990) examined rates and symptoms of anxiety across the 8- to 17-year-old age span, as well as the developmental patterns and characteristics of behavior in anxious and nonanxious community subjects. The sample was the same one previously described: 210 subjects, with 70 in each of three age groups (8-, 12-, and 17-year-olds) and equal gender representation.

Consistent with findings from other studies (Kashani and Orvaschel 1990), anxiety within this community sample was the most frequently reported DSM-III diagnosis within each age group. Though the rate for any anxiety disorder remained fairly constant, the type and content of anxiety varied with age. Fears of strangers and separation, along with somatic complaints, decreased with age, while interpersonal concerns, social fears, and anxiety about personal adequacy increased with age.

Compared with nonanxious subjects, anxious subjects manifested some interesting behavioral differences in this study. An examination of nonanxious symptoms of psychopathology showed that both groups had similar increases in depression and conduct disorder as they aged. However, anxious subjects had consistently higher levels of symptomatology at each age and for each category of pathology than did nonanxious subjects. Hence, differences were primarily quantitative in nature rather than qualitative.

Anxiety disorders had a more negative developmental consequence in the area of interpersonal relationships. While nonanxious subjects clearly improved peer relations as they aged, anxious subjects showed no improvement in this area of functioning by late adolescence. Furthermore, difficulties with family remained constant across the age span for nonanxious subjects but substantially increased with age for anxious subjects. These data indicate that anxiety disorders have their most detrimental impact on the child's interpersonal spheres of functioning.

More specific analyses were performed on anxious and nonanxious subjects across each age group. At age 8 years, anxious subjects had more psychopathological symptoms of all types than did nonanxious subjects. By age 12 years, anxious subjects also had more symptoms of psychopathology than did their nonanxious peers, as well as more difficulties in school and a poorer self-image. Finally, at age 17 years, anxious subjects had significantly more mood problems, behavioral problems, and somatic complaints and poorer self-concepts than did the nonanxious group. In sum, the data reveal that anxiety disorders affect a broad range of behaviors and that this negative impact increases with age, particularly in the interpersonal areas of the child's development.

Conclusion

There are many possible areas of explanation that remain to be explored in our attempts to account for age and gender differences in anxiety; our understanding of the developmental mechanisms underlying anxiety is incomplete. However, by combining developmental approaches with other areas of research such as epidemiology, the origins of and developmental changes in childhood anxiety can be better understood. It is important to note that such advances are dependent on improved measurement and classification systems. As suggested by Campbell (1986), more longitudinal data and research on the impact of family factors on children's fears are also needed. These will aid us in determining the degree to which childhood disorders are precursors of adult anxiety.

References

Achenbach TM: Developmental Psychopathology, 2nd Edition. New York, John Wiley, 1982

Agras WS, Chapin HH, Oliveau DC: The natural history of phobia. Arch Gen Psychiatry 26:315–317, 1972

Ainsworth MDS, Blehar M, Waters E, et al: Patterns of Attachment. Hillsdale, NJ, Lawrence Erlbaum, 1978

American Psychiatric Association: Diagnostic and Statistical Manual of Mental Disorders, 3rd Edition. Washington, DC, American Psychiatric Association, 1980

American Psychiatric Association: Diagnostic and Statistical Manual of Mental Disorders, 3rd Edition, Revised. Washington, DC, American Psychiatric Association, 1987

Barkley RA: Hyperactive Children: A Handbook for Diagnosis and Treatment. New York, Guilford, 1981

Bauer DH: An exploratory study of developmental changes in children's fears. J Child Psychol Psychiatry 17:69–74, 1976

Bowlby J: Separation: Anxiety and Anger (Attachment and Loss Series, Vol 2). New York, Basic Books, 1973

Campbell SB: Developmental issues in childhood anxiety, in Anxiety Disorders of Childhood. Edited by Gittelman R. New York, Guilford, 1986, pp 24–57

Eisenberg L: Development as a unifying concept in psychiatry. Br J Psychiatry 131:225–237, 1977

Emde R, Schmidt D: The stability of children's fears. Child Dev 49:1277–1279, 1978

Feldbaum CL, Christenson TE, O'Neal EC: An observational study of the assimilation of the newcomer to the preschool. Child Dev 51:497–507, 1980

Garber J: Classification of childhood psychopathology: a developmental perspective. Child Dev 55:30–48, 1984

Gelfand DM, Peterson L: Child Development and Psychopathology. Beverly Hills, CA, Sage, 1985

Graziano A, DeGiovanni IS, Garcia K: Behavioral treatment of children's fears: a review. Psychol Bull 86:804–830, 1979

Group for the Advancement of Psychiatry: Psychopathological Disorders in Childhood: Theoretical Considerations and a Proposed Classification. New York, Group for the Advancement of Psychiatry, 1966

Hodges KK, McKnew D, Cytryn L, et al: The Child Assessment Schedule (CAS) diagnostic interview: a report on reliability and validity. J Am Acad Child Psychiatry 21:468–473, 1982

Hoffman LW: Maternal employment: 1979. Am Psychol 34:859–865, 1979

Kashani JH, Orvaschel H: A community study of anxiety in children and adolescents. Am J Psychiatry 147:313–318, 1990

Kashani JH, Orvaschel H, Rosenberg TK, et al: Psychopathology among a community sample of children and adolescents: a developmental perspective. J Am Acad Child Adolesc Psychiatry 28:701–706, 1989

Last CG: Developmental considerations, in Issues in Diagnostic Research. Edited by Last CG, Hersen M. New York, Plenum, 1987

Last CG, Strauss CC, Francis G: Comorbidity among childhood anxiety disorders. J Nerv Ment Dis 175:726–730, 1987a

Last CG, Hersen M, Kazdin AE, et al: Comparison of DSM-III separation anxiety and overanxious disorders: demographic characteristics and patterns of comorbidity. J Am Acad Child Adolesc Psychiatry 26:527–531, 1987b

Last CG, Francis G, Hersen M, et al: Separation anxiety and school phobia: a comparison using DSM-III criteria. Am J Psychiatry 144:653–657, 1987c

Lewis M, Rosenblum LA (eds): The Origins of Fear. New York, John Wiley, 1974

McGrew WC: Aspects of social development in nursery school children with emphasis on introduction to the group, in Ethological Studies of Child Behavior. Edited by Blurton Jones N. Cambridge, England, Cambridge University Press, 1972

Miller LC, Barrett CL, Hampe E: Phobias of childhood in a prescientific era, in Child Personality and Psychopathology: Current Topics, Vol 1. Edited by Davids A. New York, John Wiley, 1974, pp 89–134

Peterson L, Burbach DJ, Chaney J: Developmental issues, in Handbook of Child Psychiatric Diagnosis. Edited by Last CG, Hersen M. New York, John Wiley, 1988, pp 463–482

Phillips L, Draguns JG, Bartlett DP: Classification of behavior disorders, in Issues in the Classification of Children. Edited by Hobbs N. San Francisco, CA, Jossey-Bass, 1975, pp 26–55

Rheingold HL, Eckerman CO: The infant separates himself from his mother. Science 168:78–83, 1970

Rutter M: The developmental psychopathology of depression: issues and perspectives, in Depression in Young People: Developmental and Clinical Perspectives. Edited by Rutter M, Izard CE, Read PB. New York, Guilford, 1986, pp 3–30

Stavrakaki C, Vargo B, Boodoosingh L, et al: The relationship between anxiety and depression in children: rating scales and clinical variables. Can J Psychiatry 32:433–439, 1987

Stayton DJ, Ainsworth MDS, Main MB: Development of separation behavior in the first year of life: protest, following, and greeting. Dev Psychol 9:213–225, 1973

Strauss CC, Last CG, Hersen M, et al: Association between anxiety and depression in children and adolescents with anxiety disorders. J Abnorm Child Psychol 16:57–68, 1988a

Strauss CC, Lease CA, Last CG, et al: Overanxious disorder: an examination of developmental differences. J Abnorm Child Psychol 16:433–443, 1988b

Wallerstein JS, Kelly JB: Surviving the Break-up—How Children and Their Parents Cope with Divorce. New York, Basic Books, 1980

Weinraub M, Lewis M: The determinants of children's responses to separation (serial no 172). Monogr Soc Res Child Dev 42(4), 1977

Chapter 14

Comorbidity

Comorbidity has been defined as "the co-occurrence of two or more disorders in the same individual at the same point in time, at a rate that is greater than would be expected by chance" (Garber 1987). The issue of comorbidity, although problematic for our system of classification, has important implications for elucidating the causal processes underlying overlapping disorders. Furthermore, the problem is particularly relevant to such distinctions as primary versus secondary disorders or internalizers versus externalizers.

However, caution must be exercised in determining actual rates of comorbidity within a population in that some covariations of disorders may simply be the result of *sampling error*; clinically referred individuals may be overrepresented in the sample if researchers sample only from among those individuals who seek treatment rather than from the general population. Yet another explanation for the co-occurrence of psychiatric disorders is *diagnostician error,* which may cause an appearance of greater-than-chance overlap. In actuality, though, this covariation may be due to the "halo effect," or the systematic tendency of clinicians to rate some symptoms as present if other particular symptoms are also present (Garber 1987). Therefore, if we can eliminate these two explanations for observed covariation, and if it is truly the case that there is a greater-than-chance covariation, then it may indeed be possible to use information about the type of covariation in order to better understand the causal processes underlying psychopathology.

Comorbidity in Adults

Although comorbidity within a child population is becoming a growing concern among researchers of childhood psychopathology, it is also frequently noted among adult population samples. In an adult community population study pertaining to exclusionary criteria of DSM-III (American Psychiatric Association 1980), Boyd et al. (1984)

concluded that there is a general tendency toward co-occurrence of disorders, such that the presence of any National Institute of Mental Health Diagnostic Interview Schedule (DIS) disorder increases the odds of having almost any other DIS disorder. This finding provides support for the clinical judgments contained in DSM-III that relate disorders to each other. This study also found that people with a dominant disorder such as major depression have a much greater likelihood of exhibiting symptoms of an excluded disorder such as panic disorder than do people without the dominant disorder. Thus, the use of exclusionary criteria in DSM-III was confirmed in this investigation.

Although Freud (1894) first proposed the differentiation of anxiety neurosis from other neurotic disorders about a century ago, the debate continues as to whether anxiety neurosis constitutes an independent disorder, distinct from other emotional illnesses (Roth and Mountjoy 1982). Particular disagreement focuses upon depression and anxiety in adults. Lewis (1938) argued that the two disorders should be unified into one concept. Similarly, Watson and Clark (1984) proposed the term "negative affectivity" to describe general emotional distress. In contrast, Roth et al. (1972) stated that the two should be considered as independent disorders. This debate has recently been applied to children and adolescents and will be discussed later in this chapter.

Overlap of DSM-III Disorders in Children

Despite considerable controversy as to the distinctiveness of specific psychiatric disorders (e.g., Lahey et al. 1980), sufficient data have been published on the frequent co-occurrence of attention-deficit disorder with hyperactivity (ADDH) and conduct disorder (CD) with oppositional disorder (OD) to justify the supradomain of "disruptive behavior disorders" as proposed by the DSM-III-R (American Psychiatric Association 1987). Researchers (Anderson et al. 1987; Reeves et al. 1987) have found significant overlap of these diagnoses in both nonreferred (6.8%) and clinical (32.5%) samples.

In the general population study by Anderson et al. (1987), the prevalence of DSM-III disorders was investigated in a sample of 792 children aged 11 years old. This was the first prevalence study to examine the extent to which DSM-III disorders overlapped. Of the 219 cases identified within the sample, 45% occurred as a single disorder, whereas 55% occurred as a combination of one or more other disorders. Eight possible categories of disorders were examined (attention-deficit disorder, OD, separation anxiety disorder, aggressive CD, over-anxious disorder, simple phobia, depression-dysthymia, and social phobia). The single disorders most frequently encountered were OD, CD, and attention-deficit disorder. The category with the fewest single disorders (*the most overlapping*) was depression-dysthymia; only 3 of the 14 children identified as depressed had a single disorder of depression-dysthymia. Each child in this group of 14 had CO or OD in addition to one or more anxious or phobic disorders. As noted by the authors, this small group of children is of considerable clinical interest since they are more likely to become clinic patients; hence, classification of their problems is obviously warranted.

In a clinical sample, Reeves et al. (1987) found that children with ADDH and children with ADDH, CD, and OD generally resembled each other in terms of sex, age at onset, psychosocial stress, and impaired cognition and achievement. These researchers found only 5.5% (6/108) to have CD and OD without concomitant ADDH, whereas 36% (39/108) of the children were found to have ADDH alone.

In a two-stage epidemiological community survey carried out by Bird et al. (1988), comorbidity of four diagnostic categories (attention-deficit disorder, affective disorder, anxiety disorder, and CD) was investigated. Findings showed that 16.6% ($n = 19$) of the children had both anxiety and affective disorders, 39.2% ($n = 36$) of the children had CD, OD, and anxiety, and 21.2% ($n = 23$) of the children had both anxiety and attention-deficit disorder. Additionally, a high degree of comorbidity among the four diagnostic groupings was apparent.

In a prospective, longitudinal design using two school-aged cohorts—one group who met DSM-III criteria for major depressive disorder (MDD), dysthymic disorder (DD), or adjustment disorder with depressed mood and one nondepressed psychiatric comparison group—Kovacs et al. (1984) found a high frequency of multiple psychiatric illnesses within the depressed group. More specifically, some type of anxiety disorder (separation anxiety, overanxious disorder, avoidant disorder, or phobic disorder) was the most common additional nonaffective diagnosis. Forty-five percent of the children who had adjustment disorder with depressed mood had additional diagnoses, most frequently anxiety (27%) or attention-deficit disorder (9%). In contrast, 79% of the children with MDD had co-occurring psychiatric disorders, with the most common being "double depression" (38%), anxiety (33%), and CD (7%). Ninety-three percent of the children with DD had co-occurring diagnosed conditions, with the most common being MDD (57%), anxiety (36%), attention-deficit disorder (14%), and CD (11%). MDD and DD did not differ significantly with respect to the likelihood of a concurrent disorder. The authors noted that the high prevalence of coexisting psychiatric illness in the depressed cohort may be due to overinclusiveness of DSM-III categories or diagnostic imprecision.

In sum, the evidence for significant comorbidity among specific childhood disorders has led to the lumping of individual diagnoses into larger categories. ADDH, CD, and OD have sufficient diagnostic overlap and so have been grouped together as "externalizing" or "behavior" disorders. Affective disorders (e.g., MDD and DD) co-occur with anxiety disorders with enough frequency that they may be considered "affective/anxiety" disorders or "internalizing" disorders (Edelbrock and Achenbach 1980). However, children who have comorbid diagnoses simultaneously from both the behavior domain and the affective/anxiety domain are more difficult to categorize.

Comorbidity of Anxiety and Depression in Children

In comparison to the adult literature, relatively few empirical investigations have examined the relationship between anxiety and depression in children and adolescents. Several of these studies are outlined below.

Bernstein and Garfinkel (1986) found that 50% of school refusers met the DSM-III criteria for both a depressive and an anxiety disorder. Also, their findings revealed that youths with both a depressive and an anxiety disorder reported higher levels of anxiety compared to those with anxiety only, depression only, or CD.

In contrast to Bernstein and Garfinkel's findings, Hershberg et al. (1982) found in their sample of 28 children with DSM-III depressive disorder and 14 children with anxiety disorder that no child with a depressive disorder had a concomitant anxiety disorder, nor did the youths who were diagnosed as having an anxiety disorder in their sample meet the DSM-III criteria for depression. (However, children with an anxiety disorder evidenced depressive symptoms and children with depressive disorder did evidence anxiety symptoms.)

Stavrakaki et al. (1987) examined the relationship between childhood anxiety and depression in the context of three adult models used to explain the complex association between the two disorders. The hypothesis of a temporal sequence between anxiety and depression emerged from their finding that depressed children were concurrently anxious, while anxious children were not concurrently depressed. Because anxiety disorder was more prevalent in the younger age group, it was hypothesized that anxious children may become depressed adolescents or adults. Hence, the present study provided evidence in support of the two disorders as separate entities in children.

Weissman et al. (1984) also investigated the relationship between anxiety and depressive disorders in children using probands of adults with 1) an MDD, 2) an MDD associated with an anxiety disorder, 3) anxiety disorder separate from MDD, and 4) a control group. The primary finding suggested that youths from probands with depression were more likely to develop a depressive disorder. Also, anxiety and MDD in the proband led to an increased risk of the children developing a psychiatric disorder, particularly an affective disorder. Thus, these findings support the utility of the concurrent diagnosis of anxiety and depressive disorders in children.

Strauss et al. (1988a) examined the relationship between anxiety and depression in a sample of 106 children and adolescents referred to an outpatient anxiety disorder clinic. Twenty-eight percent of patients with DSM-III diagnoses of anxiety disorders were found to have concurrent major depression. Compared with children who had only anxiety disorder, children with both disorders were found to be older, to have more severe anxiety symptomatology, and to be diagnosed with different rates of anxiety disorder subtypes.

Kashani and Orvaschel (1988) investigated anxiety disorders in a community sample of 150 adolescents. Seventeen percent of the adolescents met criteria for one or more anxiety diagnoses, and 8.7% were identified as being "cases" based on DSM-III criteria. The majority of the adolescents who had an anxiety disorder were noted to have at least one additional concurrent nonanxiety diagnosis. Of the 26 anxious and 12 depressed adolescents in the sample, 9 had both disorders. The comorbidity of anxiety and depression was associated with "caseness," as all 9 subjects with comorbidity were cases.

The findings discussed above regarding comorbidity of depression and anxiety reveal strong evidence for the association of the two disorders, though it is still clear that depression and anxiety may be differentiated in children. Despite the apparent association between anxiety and depression, the question still remains as to which disorder precedes the other when both occur in an individual. Seligman (1975) sheds some light on this problem through his concept of learned help-lessness. He has detected two stages in the response to danger or threat by animals and humans. When initially exposed to such influences, the individual responds with anxiety. So long as the threat continues, the anxiety persists. However, when the forces are perceived as being beyond one's control and action seems futile, depression replaces fear. Thus, Seligman regards loss of control over reinforcing factors in the environment as the central feature of clinical depression. The previously mentioned finding of Stavrakaki and his colleagues (1987) that older depressed children were concurrently anxious while younger anxious children were not concurrently depressed seems to support Seligman's contention that anxiety occurs first and depression is then superimposed on the anxiety.

Specific Comorbidity Rates of Anxiety Subtypes

Strauss et al. (1988b) examined developmental differences in a clinical sample of younger (5–11 years) and older (12–19 years) children with overanxious disorder. Comorbidity of additional diagnoses was assessed for the two groups. Results showed that younger children were significantly more likely to receive a concurrent diagnosis of separation anxiety disorder, whereas the older children more often had a concurrent diagnosis of simple phobia. Concurrent diagnosis of agoraphobia and panic disorder was present only in the older group.

Kashani and Orvaschel (1990) investigated comorbidity among subtypes of anxiety disorders in a clinical sample of 100 children. Twenty-one of the 100 children were considered to have "severe" anxiety (based on symptom report by both the parent and child), 48 children were considered to have a "possible" anxiety (based on symptom report by only one informant), and 31 children had no anxiety diagnosis. Thirteen of the 21 severely anxious children were diagnosed as having more than one type of anxiety disorder (based on the Diagnostic Interview for Children and Adolescents), and 5 of the 21 had all three possible anxiety disorders (separation anxiety, phobia, and over-anxious disorder).

In a study by Last et al. (1987c) investigating the use of DSM-III criteria for differentiating separation anxiety disorder and school phobic disorder, data on concurrent anxiety disorders were presented. One-half of the children in both the separation anxiety disorder group ($n = 48$) and school phobia group ($n = 19$) met DSM-III criteria for at least one additional anxiety diagnosis. The most frequently occurring anxiety diagnosis for both of the groups was overanxious disorder (46% of the children with separation anxiety disorder and 37% of the children with school phobia). Also, children with separation anxiety disorder were more likely to have a concurrent psychiatric disorder than were the children with school phobia ($P < .05$).

Last et al. (1987b) compared separation anxiety and overanxious disorders along the dimensions of demographic characteristics and patterns of comorbidity. Over 50% of the overanxious disorder group ($n = 26$) met criteria for at least one additional anxiety diagnosis, compared with only one child in the separation anxiety group ($n = 22$). More specifically, the overanxious disorder group was significantly more likely to have an additional diagnosis of simple phobia than was the group that had no concurrent diagnosis of simple phobia.

Finally, comorbidity among childhood anxiety disorders was the focus of another investigation by Last et al. (1987a). Seventy-three children and adolescents (aged 5–18 years) were evaluated with a structured diagnostic interview to examine patterns of comorbidity. Again, children with a primary diagnosis of separation anxiety disorder were the least likely to receive a concurrent anxiety diagnosis (58%). The most common concurrent disorder for the separation anxiety disorder group was overanxious disorder (33%). However, those children with a primary diagnosis of overanxious disorder were most likely to have a coexisting diagnosis of social phobia (36%) or OD (36%). Overall, findings from this study identify relatively distinct groups of anxious children and support the recent DSM-III revisions.

The research cited above clearly documents the high prevalence of comorbid behavior associated with anxiety disorders both in the general population and in clinical samples. Although comorbidity is a serious problem for our system of classification, it can also provide a unique opportunity for examining questions pertaining to childhood psychopathology. The complexity of the condition enables health care workers to obtain more detailed information as to the patient's disorder. This may lead to more diverse options and ultimately improved patient care. However, treatment plans should consider the *whole* person; treatment of one disorder while ignoring a co-occurring disorder is clearly both frustrating and suboptimal.

References

American Psychiatric Association: Diagnostic and Statistical Manual of Mental Disorders, 3rd Edition. Washington, DC, American Psychiatric Association, 1980

American Psychiatric Association: Diagnostic and Statistical Manual of Mental Disorders, 3rd Edition, Revised. Washington, DC, American Psychiatric Association, 1987

Anderson JC, Williams S, McGee R, et al: DSM-III disorders in preadolescent children. Arch Gen Psychiatry 44:69–76, 1987

Bernstein GA, Garfinkel BB: School phobia: the overlap of affective and anxiety disorders. J Am Acad Child Psychiatry 25:235–241, 1986

Bird HR, Canino G, Rubio-Stipec M, et al: Estimates of the prevalence of childhood maladjustment in a community survey in Puerto Rico. Arch Gen Psychiatry 45:1120–1126, 1988

Boyd JH, Burke JD, Gruenberg E, et al: Exclusion criteria of DSM-III. Arch Gen Psychiatry 41:983–989, 1984

Edelbrock L, Achenbach TM: A topology of child behavior profile patterns: distribution and correlates for disturbed children aged 6–16. J Abnorm Child Psychol 8:441–470, 1980

Freud S: The justification for detaching from neurasthenia a particular syndrome: the anxiety-neurosis (1894), in Collected Papers, Vol 1. Edited by Jones E. London, Hogarth Press, 1924, pp 76–106

Garber J: Comorbidity with depression in children: the validity of the primary versus secondary distinction. Paper presented at the annual meeting of the American Academy of Child and Adolescent Psychiatry, Washington, DC, October 1987

Hershberg SS, Carlson GA, Cantwell DP, et al: Anxiety and depressive disorders in psychiatrically disturbed children. J Clin Psychiatry 43:358–361, 1982

Kashani JH, Orvaschel H: Anxiety disorders in mid-adolescence: a community sample. Am J Psychiatry 145:960–964, 1988

Kashani JH, Orvaschel H: A community study of anxiety in children and adolescents. Am J Psychiatry 147:313–318, 1990

Kovacs M, Feinberg TL, Crouse-Novak MA, et al: Depressive disorders in childhood, I: a longitudinal prospective study of characteristics and recovery. Arch Gen Psychiatry 41:229–237, 1984

Lahey BD, Green KD, Forehand R: On the independence of rating of hyperactivity, conduct problems, and attention deficits in children: a multiple regression. 1980

Last CG, Strauss CC, Francis G: Comorbidity among childhood anxiety disorders. J Nerv Ment Dis 175:726–730, 1987a

Last CG, Hersen M, Kazdin AE, et al: Comparison of DSM-III separation anxiety and overanxious disorders: demographic characteristics and patterns of comorbidity. J Am Acad Child Adolesc Psychiatry 26:527–531, 1987b

Last CG, Francis G, Hersen M, et al: Separation anxiety and school phobia: a comparison using DSM III criteria. Am J Psychiatry 144:635–657, 1987c

Lewis A: States of depression: their clinical and etiological differentiation. Br Med J 2:875–878, 1938

Reeves JC, Werry J, Elkind GS, et al: Attention deficit, conduct, oppositional and anxiety disorders in children, II: clinical characteristics. J Am Acad Child Adolesc Psychiatry 26:144–155, 1987

Roth M, Mountjoy CQ: The distinction between anxiety states and depressive disorders, in Handbook of Affective Disorders. Edited by Paykel ES. New York, Guilford, 1982, pp 70–92

Roth M, Gurney C, Garside RF, et al: Studies in the classification of affective disorders: the relationship between anxiety states and depressive illness, I. Br J Psychiatry 121:147–161, 1972

Seligman M: Helplessness: On Depression, Development and Death. San Francisco, CA, WH Freeman, 1975

Stavrakaki C, Vargo B, Boodoosingh L, et al: The relationship between anxiety and depression in children: rating scales and clinical variables. Can J Psychiatry 32:433–439, 1987

Strauss CC, Last CG, Hersen M, et al: Association between anxiety and depression in children and adolescents with anxiety disorders. J Abnorm Child Psychol 16:57–68, 1988a

Strauss CC, Lease CA, Last CG, et al: Overanxious disorder: an examination of development differences. J Abnorm Child Psychol 16:433–443, 1988b

Watson D, Clark LA: Negative affectivity: the disposition to experience aversive emotional states. Psychol Bull 96:465–490, 1984

Weissman MM, Leckman J, Merikangas KR, et al: Depression and anxiety disorders in parents and children. Arch Gen Psychiatry 41:845–852, 1984

Chapter 15

Treatment

"**A**dults seem to minimize the importance of children's fears and to view such fears as a common, expected, transitory and thus not particularly serious part of normal development" (Graziano 1978, p. 283). This popular viewpoint that fears and anxieties in childhood are a "normal" part of development is a primary reason for the paucity of literature pertaining to treatment of childhood anxiety disorders. Only when the child's emotional state is extremely severe and the illness is of significant duration does the child receive attention from mental health professionals.

Discussion of the treatment of anxiety disorders is limited by the lack of an empirically based and generally accepted definition of childhood anxiety disorders (Carlson et al. 1986). Considerable work is needed before the conclusion can be made that DSM-III-R criteria (American Psychiatric Association 1987) for the various anxiety disorders have scientific merit. Furthermore, researchers are currently in a period of transition in the development of specific treatment approaches; different methods generally do not differ in their efficacy (Bloch 1982). For this reason, it is recommended that psychiatrists assess individual cases at multiple conceptual levels for the purpose of establishing the most appropriate treatment program.

In this chapter, we will individually examine four of the most prevalent treatment programs: 1) pharmacotherapy, 2) behavioral therapy, 3) family therapy, and 4) psychoanalytic therapy. In actual clinical practice, however, several different treatment approaches are often used simultaneously to suit the needs of the individual patient. We will then briefly discuss the treatment literature pertaining to the specific anxiety subtypes of overanxious disorder, separation anxiety disorder, and obsessive-compulsive disorder.

Psychopharmacology

One of the critical dimensions for defining and measuring anxiety is visceral and somatic activation (Lang 1984). This usually involves sympathetic arousal and results in the psychophysiological symptoms associated with anxiety. Depending on the individual, however, response patterns vary; anxious patients usually display a disproportionate degree of control and autonomic arousal in response to disturbing stimuli, and they have an inability to adapt to a changing environment. When relaxed, anxious patients exhibit an increase in skin conductance, as well as increases in heart rate and blood pressure.

Drugs prescribed for the treatment of anxiety disorders fall into five classes: neuroleptics, psychostimulants, antihistamines, anxiolytics, and antidepressants.

Neuroleptics

For decades after their introduction, neuroleptics such as chlorpromazine were called tranquilizers (Gittelman and Koplewicz 1986). But it eventually became apparent that their sedating and anxiolytic actions were totally independent of one another. Controlled studies of their use in treating anxiety disorders of childhood are lacking. Three placebo-controlled studies of neuroleptics have been reported for inpatient groups (Freedman et al. 1955; Garfield et al. 1962; Lucas and Pasley 1969). None of the studies supported the use of neuroleptics for relief of anxiety disorders.

A review by Gittelman-Klein (1978) noted that all neuroleptic studies pertaining to childhood and adolescent anxiety states were unsatisfactory because of the sample inadequacies (mixing psychotic children with children who had behavioral disorders) and the imprecise nature of the patient groups. Given neuroleptics' potential for restricting cognitive functioning or causing tardive dyskinesia, many feel that the use of these agents as treatment should be restricted except for the most severe anxiety cases.

Psychostimulants

Contrary to what one would expect from psychostimulants, amphetamines have been reported and observed to be useful in relieving anxiety and stimulating overly inhibited neurotic children (e.g., Fish

1968). However, other studies observed that hyperactive children who also had overanxious disorder responded adversely on cognitive tests to methylphenidate (Swanson et al. 1978). Hence, there is no conclusive evidence that stimulants are effective in children whose *primary* clinical problem is anxiety.

Antihistamines

This group includes diphenhydramine, hydroxyzine, and promethazine. Again, the evidence for the use of these agents in the treatment of anxiety disorders is lacking. However, uncontrolled studies of mixed diagnostic groups have claimed that diphenhydramine (Benadryl) and hydroxyzine (Atarax) modified anxiety symptoms (Effron and Freedman 1953; Fish 1968).

Anxiolytics

Also formerly called tranquilizers, these were renamed "minor tranquilizers" when the major tranquilizers were introduced. Sedation is the most well known effect of this class of drugs. Barbiturates have been replaced by the benzodiazepines because of their greater margin of safety (Gittelman and Koplewicz 1986). Compared to the literature on adults, there are few published reports of the effects of benzodiazepines on children who were treated primarily for anxiety disorders. Clinical experience suggests that stimulating and paradoxical effects may occur because of disinhibition, despite the fact that children tolerate these agents without difficulty (McDermott et al. 1989). Benzodiazepines may be useful for children whose separation anxiety has cleared with tricyclic medication but who are still troubled with situational and anticipatory anxiety.

Antidepressants

The use of antidepressants in anxiety disorders is based on the belief that anxiety is a form of depression (Gittelman and Koplewicz 1986).

Tricyclic antidepressants and monoamine oxidase inhibitors are the two major groups of antidepressants. Tricyclic antidepressants, particularly imipramine, have been very effective in the treatment of anxiety disorders in children and adolescents (McDermott et al. 1989). Furthermore, since imipramine relieved adult panic anxiety and since panic anxiety is considered to be a pathological variant of separation anxiety, then it follows that imipramine might be useful in treating children with separation anxiety (Klein 1964).

In a study by Rabiner and Klein (1969), a clinical trial was conducted using imipramine in children who had school phobia (since their phobic disorder is often the consequence of separation anxiety disorder). Eighty-five percent of the children returned to school. Gittelman-Klein and Klein (1971) found that imipramine was significantly superior to placebo, both in facilitating anxiety symptoms and in inducing return to school. Unfortunately, many side effects are associated with the tricyclics, including seizures (Preskorn et al. 1983), changes in cardiac functioning, and even deaths due to overdosage.

In sum, clinical reports investigating pharmacotherapy have many methodological limitations, such as a variable length of treatment with no attempt to evaluate treatment outcome at some fixed point (Gittelman and Koplewicz 1986). However, evidence based on the literature reveals that, of the various agents, tricyclics may have a powerful role in the early management of severe anxiety disorders. Additionally, the clinical reports suggest that benzodiazepines may also be quite effective in the treatment of childhood anxiety disorders. However, at this time, the evidence for antianxiety pharmacological treatment is inconclusive.

Behavioral Therapy

Behavioral theory assumes that certain stimuli evoke naturally occurring innate behaviors that form the foundation on which learned or conditioned behaviors are built. Although excellent reviews of behavioral treatment have been published (see Kratochwill and Morris 1985; Morris and Kratochwill 1985), this section will describe the five primary behavioral methods used by clinicians today: systematic desensitization, flooding and implosive therapy, modeling, operant conditioning, and cognitive-behavioral strategies.

Systematic Desensitization

With this approach, the child is presented with the anxiety-inducing situation. However, safety is ensured in this controlled setting, and hence there is no gain in avoiding the situation. According to Wolpe

(1958), the anxiety response is inhibited by pairing the anxiety-producing stimulus with an incompatible response; this paired response is typically relaxation, although other anxiety-antagonistic responses can be used. Graduated imagined stimuli, as well as relaxation, have been used to treat such problems as tics, anorexia nervosa, phobia of loud noises, and phobia of dogs, to name a few (see Hatzenbuehler and Schroeder 1978). In the example of dog phobia, desensitization techniques require the child to be exposed to dogs in a graduated fashion (i.e., first to small dogs and then to large dogs, first with and then without an adult's presence) until the fear is extinguished.

Flooding and Implosion

Like desensitization, flooding and implosive therapy involves exposing the child to anxiety-eliciting stimuli. This approach, however, entails exposing the child to stimuli that elicit high levels of anxiety and forcing the child to remain in the situation until the anxiety response is extinguished (e.g., Stampfl and Levis 1967). Implosive therapy is based on learning theory placed within a psychodynamic framework; Stampfl and Levis (1967) propose that defense mechanisms are the means through which anxiety-producing stimuli are avoided. Hence, defense mechanisms are reinforced and maintained. The process consists of selecting certain cues derived from present behavior, along with psychodynamic themes such as rejection, dependency, and anality. The therapist then requests the child to react with genuine emotion to scenes generated from the cues. Finally, the scenes are presented in terms of the degree of associated avoidance. This is repeated until all the anxiety has been extinguished. Flooding (Marks 1975) is a similar technique; however, exposure is limited to stimuli *directly* associated with the anxiety rather than to psychodynamic elements, as in implosion therapy. Prior to these therapeutic tactics, a successful outcome requires proper preparation and sufficient cooperation of both the child and parent. Great care should be taken to ensure that the welfare of the patient is protected.

Modeling

Three types of modeling have been investigated in anxiety research: symbolic modeling, live models, and participant modeling. Although research on the effectiveness of these three types of modeling reveals that participant modeling is superior to the others, a review of the literature suggests that conclusions in this area remain tentative (Graziano et al. 1979).

Symbolic modeling (noted as the least effective method) enables the therapist to have control over the events taking place; hence, method variance is minimized. In contrast, live-modeling methodology consists of children watching a "live" model interact with a feared object. In participant modeling, the child watches a model go through a gradual approach sequence—first, the child watches the model perform the desired actions and then the child imitates the model. Finally, the child performs the responses without the assistance of the model. This method is commonly referred to as "contact desensitization" (Carlson et al. 1986). Graziano et al. (1979) recommended that the therapist consider the enhanced efficacy of modeling when paired with direct exposure to the phobic stimulus (e.g., participant modeling) in choosing a given type of modeling. Other considerations include the characteristics of the model and the number of models presented (Carlson et al. 1986).

Operant Conditioning

In operant conditioning, the child is provided with reinforcement for either 1) not avoiding or 2) avoiding the fear-eliciting situation (McDermott et al. 1989). For example, in treating a child with dog phobia, praise would be given to the child at each step of approach, culminating in a reward when final success was achieved. A well-designed systematic study of preschool children who feared darkness was performed by Lietenberg and Callahan (1973) in order to evaluate the effectiveness of reinforced practice. At posttest, results showed that the children exposed to the reinforcement were willing to remain in the dark significantly longer than were children from the control group. However, the study should be interpreted cautiously because of the limited number of subjects and the inability to quantify each subject's degree of fearfulness. Although many positive outcomes have been described in operant-conditioning studies, few published studies have adequately assessed the usefulness of this procedure (Carlson et al. 1986).

Cognitive-Behavioral Model

The cognitive-behavioral model encompasses the relationships of cognitions and behavior to the affective state of the individual and to the interaction of that individual within his or her social context (Kendall et al. 1988). This model is best illustrated by the work of Kanfer et al. (1975), who utilized self-control procedures to increase tolerance of the dark in fearful kindergarten-aged children. Forty-five children were assigned to one of three groups (two treatment and one control). The children were given one of three types of self-statements to rehearse. In the competence group, children used positive self-statements such as "I am brave boy (girl). I can take care of myself in the dark." In the second condition (stimulus), children practiced statements such as "The dark is a fun place to be." The third, neutral group was asked to repeat a distracting nursery rhyme. Dependent measures included two trials measuring the length of time the child could remain in a darkened room and two trials determining the level of illumination chosen by the child in the experimenter's absence. At posttest, both treatment groups out-performed the control group in dark-tolerance measures on the first trial and all groups showed increased tolerance on the second trial, with the competence group showing the most improvement. On the illumination measure, the treatment groups tolerated lower levels than did the other two groups on the first trial; both treatment groups showed greater tolerance on the second trial.

Generalizability of the results with the children in this study to clinically anxious populations, however, is limited. The few studies published in the area of cognitive-behavioral applications have focused on the prevention of nighttime fears, fear of dental procedures, test and public speaking anxiety, and clinical case studies (Kendall et al. 1988). Further research in this area seems warranted based on the positive results described above.

Family Therapy

This type of treatment suggests that working with the family system is the most effective way to alleviate the anxiety experienced by the child (McDermott et al. 1989). The child's symptom is first conceptualized as an individual problem and then reformulated in terms of how the child's disorder coincides with the family style and behavior. After the therapist observes the child in the context of the family, family dynamics are examined for dysfunctional patterns. Concepts such as triangulation and scapegoating are conceptualized in individual terms. The primary goal of family intervention is to replace dysfunctional anxiety-producing repetitive patterns with new, more functional patterns (McDermott et al. 1989). More specifically, the therapist investigates information at a variety of levels: 1) factual answers given by the informants, 2) perceptions of different family members, and 3) behavior. The therapist may even request an enactment of anxiety-eliciting situations. The family members learn to understand themselves by looking at themselves through this inquiry. The therapist also searches for resources of family competence and ways in which to mobilize these resources therapeutically.

Psychoanalytic Psychotherapy

The basic tenet behind psychoanalytic theory is that anxiety disorders are caused by unconscious conflicts related to sexual and aggressive drives (McDermott et al. 1989). Under certain conditions, these conflicts can no longer be repressed adequately and the symptoms of overt anxiety appear. Intensive individual psychoanalytic psychotherapy places great emphasis on interpretation of, or rendering conscious, that which is unconscious or preconscious. Psychotherapy involves three major phases: the initial phase, the middle phase, and the termination phase.

During the first phase, a therapeutic alliance between the therapist and the child is fostered. Once the child has some understanding of why he or she is seeing a therapist, the first goal is to enable the child to experience a nonjudgmental, understanding response to his or her behavior (Lewis 1986). The focus of the middle phase is an interpretation of the transference. The child's play is part of the association process in the context of therapy, a type of "free association." The therapist's task is to keep the material flowing, focusing more and more on underlying fears and anxieties as they emerge through the child's play. Simultaneously, the child talks, exhibits mannerisms, and portrays attitudes that enable the therapist to form associative threads. Hence, therapy is usually directed in such a way that the child is hardly aware that treatment is taking place. During the phase of termination, issues such as separation, reactions to loss, and so forth are explored.

This period ideally includes achievement of goals such as reduced anxiety, improved self-esteem, and increased frustration tolerance. Hopefully, the child will have gained a better understanding of himself or herself. The primary aim of psychoanalysis is not merely to relieve anxiety symptoms, but to bring about a lasting change in the underlying personality structure.

Treatment Associated With Separation Anxiety

In 1917, Freud discussed the primary importance of separation from mother as the origin of anxiety: "A child is first afraid of strange people . . . because the stranger's face is not mother's familiar beloved face" (Freud 1917, p. 407). Freud proposed that the prototypical separation from mother occurs at birth and that "the affect of anxiety repeats the early impression of the act of birth." Psychodynamic psychotherapy for a child with separation anxiety is thus centered around an avoidance of the oedipal conflict (with mother) and a regression to the earlier development issue of separation and individuation from the mother.

The ubiquity of separation anxiety suggests that this phase in a child's life may be an evolved adaptive response enhancing the reproductive success of the species (Thyer and Sowers-Hoag 1988). Many features characteristic of separation anxiety disorder differ in quantity but not quality from behaviors displayed by all children. In other words, separation anxiety disorder may represent an exaggeration or extension of earlier, natural developmental phenomena. Although the disorder is likely to develop following a significant stressor in the life of the child, this vulnerability is not specific to separation anxiety disorder (Thyer and Sowers-Hoag 1988).

Phenomenologically, separation anxiety in children has been related to panic disorder experienced by adult agoraphobic patients. Gittelman-Klein and Klein (1971) noted that a large proportion of adult agoraphobic patients had a childhood history of severe separation anxiety and that their initial response to panic was characterized by clinging, dependent behavior. They postulated that these adult patients' biological process regulating the anxiety caused by separation was disrupted. Since panic attacks in the agoraphobic patient have been shown to respond significantly to antidepressants (e.g., imipramine), it was suggested that imipramine would be useful in relieving separation anxiety. Imipramine was thus tried in school-phobic children and was found to be superior to placebo.

Reports of systematic behavioral treatment of severe separation anxiety first appeared almost 30 years ago, yet the literature in this area remains sparse (Thyer and Sowers-Hoag 1988). Most studies are narrative case reports, and only a very few involve the use of single subject research designs. Hence, the *experimental* evidence for the efficacy of behavior therapy for separation anxiety disorder is nonexistent. However, a review of the literature also reveals that behavior therapy as a treatment approach to separation anxiety disorder is considerably superior to other interventions such as psychoanalytic and supportive therapy (Thyer and Sowers-Hoag 1988).

Treatment Associated With Overanxious Disorder

The primary characteristic of overanxious disorder is the lack of focus on a specific situation or object (Strauss 1988). Overanxious disorder in children is similar to the adult-onset diagnosis of generalized anxiety disorder, but it is unknown whether the first is the developmental precursor of the latter.

Although overanxious children are frequently referred for clinical outpatient services, no reports to date have been published regarding effective treatments for children and adolescents with overanxious disorder (Strauss 1988). However, hypotheses for such treatment have been developed based on the literature pertaining to treatment for generalized anxiety disorder in adults (e.g., anxiety management). Because of the lack of evidence supporting a particular intervention program for overanxious disorder, a treatment package modeled after the adult anxiety management program has been developed (Strauss 1988). This therapy integrates several approaches: 1) relaxation techniques (muscle relaxation and visual imagery of pleasant scenes), 2) positive self-statements, 3) a home-based token economy program to reward nonanxious behavior, and 4) cognitive control in which children and adolescents engage in coping strategies to achieve relaxation. These techniques have also been employed successfully in children and adolescents with specific fears or phobias (see Carlson et al. 1986).

Treatment Associated With
Obsessive-Compulsive Disorder

Lack of research on the treatment of obsessive-compulsive disorder is not surprising given the disorder's low prevalence rate in children (fewer than 2% of child psychiatric populations) (Hollingsworth et al. 1980). Nevertheless, this disorder (in both children and adults) has been of major interest to researchers and a challenge to psychiatrists wishing to treat it effectively.

Despite the lack of success with the majority of pharmacological interventions (e.g., neuroleptics, lithium carbonate, the benzodiazepines), the new tricyclic antidepressant clomipramine has been consistently effective in treating obsessive-compulsive disorder in children, adolescents, and adults (Ananth 1983). Flament et al. (1985) showed that clomipramine was significantly more effective than placebo in controlling the symptoms of obsessive-compulsive behavior in adolescents.

It is now clear, however, that the most efficient treatment program incorporates one or more behavioral techniques. Treatment in this area has included aversion relief, graded exposure, satiation, systematic desensitization, modeling, and positive reinforcement, to name only a few. It is important to note that virtually all of the behavioral treatment reports on children with obsessive-compulsive disorder have included family participation. Hence, behavioral therapy is maximally effective only when combined with family therapy. However, there are no investigations to date comparing drug trials and behavioral treatments in children.

The most successful behavioral treatment utilized thus far for the treatment of obsessive-compulsive disorder has been response prevention. Stanley (1980) reported on the use of this method in treating a complex set of rituals (e.g., incessant pillow fluffing, singing specific nursery rhymes) exhibited by an 8-year-old girl. Treatment consisted of working with the family to ensure that the child engaged in the ritualistic behaviors only once at any given time and that the ritual gradually be extinguished. This response prevention technique was successful in that the rituals disappeared within 2 weeks, with no recurrences reported during a 1-year follow-up.

In sum, children's fears are not always transitory and simply a "normal" part of their early years. The first step in treatment appears to be determining whether a child has situational anxiety symptoms or chronic anxiety. Identification of a specific type of anxiety follows, along with appropriate treatment programs. Currently, more research is needed on the topic of specific anxiety disorders among different age groups. Pending the development of specific treatment techniques, however, it is recommended that the therapist conceptualize the symptoms on various levels in order to find the best program for each child's individual needs.

References

American Psychiatric Association: Diagnostic and Statistical Manual of Mental Disorders, 3rd Edition, Revised. Washington, DC, American Psychiatric Association, 1987

Ananth J: Clomipramine in obsessive-compulsive disorder: a review. Psychosomatics 24:723–727, 1983

Bloch S: Psychotherapy, in Recent Advances in Clinical Psychiatry, Vol 4. Edited by Granville-Grossman K. Edinburgh, Churchill Livingstone, 1982, pp 25–45

Carlson CL, Figueroa RG, Lahey BB: Behavior therapy for childhood anxiety disorders, in Anxiety Disorders of Childhood. Edited by Gittelman R. New York, Guilford, 1986, pp 204–232

Effron AJ, Freedman AM: The treatment of behavior disorders in children with Benadryl. J Pediatrics 42:261–266, 1953

Fish B: Drug use in psychiatric disorders in children. Am J Psychiatry 124:31–36, 1968

Flament MF, Rapoport JL, Murphy D, et al: Clomipramine treatment of childhood obsessive-compulsive disorder: a double-blind controlled study. Arch Gen Psychiatry 42:977–983, 1985

Freedman AA, Effron AS, Bender L: Pharmacotherapy in children with psychiatric illness. J Nerv Ment Dis 22:479–486, 1955

Freud S: Introductory lectures on psychoanalysis. Lecture 25: anxiety (1917), in The Standard Edition of the Complete Psychological Works of Sigmund Freud, Vol 16. Translated and edited by Strachey J. London, Hogarth Press, 1963, pp 392–411

Garfield SL, Helper MM, Wilcott RC, et al: Effects of chlorpromazine on behavior in emotionally disturbed children. J Nerv Ment Dis 135:147–154, 1962

Gittelman-Klein R: Psychopharmacological treatment of anxiety disorders, mood disorders and Tourette's disorder in children, in Psychopharmacology: A Generation of Progress. Edited by Lipton MA, Dimascio A, Killan KF. New York, Raven, 1978, pp 1471–1480

Gittelman-Klein R, Klein DF: Controlled imipramine treatment of school phobia. Arch Gen Psychiatry 25:204–207, 1971

Gittelman R, Koplewicz HS: Pharmacotherapy of childhood anxiety disorders, in Anxiety Disorders of Childhood. Edited by Gittelman R. New York, Guilford, 1986, pp 188–203

Graziano AM: Behavior therapy, in Handbook of Treatment of Mental Disorders in Childhood and Adolescence. Edited by Wolman BB, Egan J, Russ AO. Englewood Cliffs, NJ, Prentice-Hall, 1978

Graziano AM, DeGiovanni I, Garcia K: Behavioral treatment of child's fears: a review. Psychol Bull 56:804–830, 1979

Hatzenbuehler LC, Schroeder HE: Desensitization procedures in the treatment of childhood disorders. Psychol Bull 85:331–844, 1978

Hollingsworth CE, Tanguey PE, Grossman L, et al: Long-term outcome of obsessive-compulsive disorder in childhood. J Am Acad Child Psychiatry 19:134–144, 1980

Kanfer FH, Karoly P, Newman A: Reduction of children's fear of the dark by competence-related and situational threat-related verbal cries. J Consult Clin Psychol 43:251–258, 1975

Kendall PC, Howard BL, Epps J: The anxious child: cognitive-behavioral treatment strategies. Behav Modif 12:281–310, 1988

Klein DF: Delineation of two drug-responsive anxiety syndromes. Psychopharmacologia 5:397–408, 1964

Kratochwill TR, Morris RJ: Conceptual and methodological issues in the behavioral assessment and treatment of children's fears and phobias. School Psychology Review 14:94–107, 1985

Lang PJ: State-of-the-art conference reviews new developments in characterizing, treating anxiety. Hosp Community Psychiatry 35:9–10, 1984

Lewis M: Principles of intensive individual psychoanalytic psychotherapy for childhood anxiety disorders, in Anxiety Disorders of Childhood. Edited by Gittelman R. New York, Guilford, 1986, pp 233–255

Lietenberg H, Callahan EJ: Reinforced practice and reduction of different kinds of fears in adults and children. Behav Res Ther 11:19–30, 1973

Lucas AR, Pasley FC: Psychoactive drugs in the treatment of emotionally disturbed children: haloperidol and diazepam. Compr Psychiatry 10:376–386, 1969

Marks IM: Behavioral treatments of phobic and obsessive-compulsive disorders: a critical appraisal, in Progress in Behavior Modification, Vol 1. Edited by Hersen M, Eisler RM, Miller PM. New York, Academic, 1975, pp 65–158

McDermott JF Jr, Werry J, Petti T, et al: Anxiety disorders of childhood or adolescence, in Treatments of Psychiatric Disorders: A Task Force Report of the American Psychiatric Association, Vol 1. Washington, DC, American Psychiatric Association, 1989, pp 401–446

Morris RJ, Kratochwill TR: Behavioral treatment of children's fears and phobias. School Psychology Review 14:84–93, 1985

Preskorn SH, Weller EB, Weller RA, et al: Plasma levels of imipramine and adverse effects in children. Am J Psychiatry 140:1332–1335, 1983

Rabiner CJ, Klein DF: Imipramine treatment of school phobia. Compr Psychiatry 10:387–390, 1969

Stampfl TG, Levis DJ: Essentials of implosive therapy: a learning-theory-based psychodynamic behavioral therapy. J Abnorm Psychol 72:496–503, 1967

Stanley L: Treatment of ritualistic behavior in an eight-year-old girl by response prevention: a case report. J Child Psychol Psychiatry 21:85–90, 1980

Strauss CC: Behavioral assessment and treatment of overanxious disorder in children and adolescents. Behav Modif 12:234–251, 1988

Swanson J, Kinsbourne M, Roberts W, et al: Time-response analysis of the effect of stimulant medication on the learning ability of children referred for hyperactivity. Pediatrics 61:21–24, 1978

Thyer BA, Sowers-Hoag KM: Behavior therapy for separation anxiety disorder. Behav Modif 12:205–233, 1988

Wolpe J: Psychotherapy by Reciprocal Inhibition. Stanford, CA, Stanford University Press, 1958

Chapter 16

Natural History of Anxiety Disorders

*T*he study of the natural history of childhood disorders, i.e., their course and outcome, is a very important area of research. It provides knowledge about predictive factors and prognosis, and their relationship to adult psychopathology. Literature on the natural history of anxiety disorders can be generally divided into three investigational strategies: 1) the relationship between childhood and adult-onset anxiety, 2) follow-up studies of children with anxiety disorders, and 3) retrospective studies of adults with anxiety disorders. Each of these strategies will be discussed separately.

Relationship Between Childhood and Adult Anxiety

The research linking childhood anxiety disorders with adult psychopathology suffers from definitional and methodological difficulties. Earlier studies aggregated anxiety syndrome and emotional disturbances (Rutter and Garmezy 1983); thus, anxiety was only one of an entire class of symptoms that were in reality distinct from another aggregate class of symptoms—behavior disorders. In Rutter et al.'s Isle of Wight study (1981) children with "emotional" disorders at age 11 years were twice as likely as other youngsters to have psychiatric disorders as adolescents. These children retained the same diagnoses, and none was found to have developed conduct disorder by age 15 years.

Studies on shyness and fears show that they are relatively stable phenomena (Emde and Schmidt 1978; MacFarlane et al. 1954). Richman et al. (1982) reported that fears in 3-year-old children were associated with "neurotic" disorders at 5-year follow-up, but that these children were not at risk for any other psychiatric disorder at age 8 years. An earlier study (Morris et al. 1954), however, reported a more optimistic outcome for 34 children treated for shy and withdrawn behaviors.

Generalizations regarding the implications of childhood anxiety disorders for illness in later life are not without ambiguity. Orvaschel and Weissman (1986) suggest that diagnostic specificity cannot be projected from childhood; however, they do endorse a general relationship between childhood and adult anxiety disorders. Rutter (1986) advances the notion of temporal contiguity and cautiously asserts diagnostic consistency from childhood through adulthood. He postulates that psychiatric disorders, if they are to recur in later life, are consistent with the type of disorder exhibited in early life. That is, those children and adolescents with a history of anxiety disorders will again present as adults with an anxiety-centered pathology. This developmental continuity is most consistently seen in obsessive-compulsive disorder (Zeitlen 1983).

Agoraphobia and panic disorder in adults may be sequelae to childhood separation anxiety disorder. Klein (1981) inferred a functional relationship from retrospective reports of adults so afflicted, who presented with separation anxiety as children. A prospective study by Rutter (1985) suggests but does not conclusively explicate an association between juvenile-onset separation anxiety and subsequent adult panic disorder or agoraphobia.

Follow-up Studies

Most of the follow-up studies (Emde and Schmidt 1978; MacFarlane et al. 1954; Richman et al. 1982; Rutter et al. 1981) discussed above were conducted in England among children who were drawn from the general population. A more recent study (Fischer et al. 1984) in the United States did not find a continuity of dysfunction from childhood to adult anxiety disorders. However, these authors derived their data from the rating scales filled out by the parents and did not perform direct clinical assessment.

A number of researchers have studied the relationship between early temperaments characteristic of social inhibition in children and the later development of anxiety disorders (Kagan 1988; Kagan et al. 1987; Reznik et al. 1986). These findings support the notion that social inhibition as a temperamental characteristic in children may represent a premorbid feature of childhood anxiety disorder and predispose to later anxious symptomatology (Klein and Last 1989). Some supportive evidence for this theory is provided by Rosenbaum and his colleagues

(1988), who studied a small sample of 2- to 7-year-old children of adults with panic disorder and found that these children had more social inhibition than did children of normal adults. However, this difference was not found among children of depressed adults.

Follow-up studies from the clinical population of children with anxiety disorders primarily involve children with school phobia and are marred by a lack of systematic diagnostic assessment (Klein and Last 1989). Berg and colleagues (1976) in a 3-year follow-up study of 100 previously hospitalized children found that those with adjustment problems were worse at 3 years than at 1 year postdischarge. Five of these children developed agoraphobia, half had poor school attendance, and 50–70% had other symptomatology. Children with higher IQs had worse outcome (Berg et al. 1976). Other studies (Roberts 1975; Weiss and Burke 1970) also reported similar results.

In a more recent study by Berg and Jackson (1985), high IQ predicted more positive outcome. Fourteen percent of the children in this study still required outpatient treatment 10 years after their discharge from the hospital, and 5% required rehospitalization during the interim. Those patients who received treatment before age 14 years had a more favorable outcome. However, this study has many methodological drawbacks, among them the lack of controls and standardized interviews.

Many investigators have studied outpatient populations of children with school phobia (e.g., Coolidge et al. 1964; Miller et al. 1972; Rodriguez et al. 1959; Waldron 1976). All have shown a better outcome among younger children and a significant number of adjustment problems at follow-up.

A more recent study (Flakierska et al. 1988) reported on 15-year to 20-year follow-up of 35 school-phobic children first identified between 7 and 12 years of age by a survey of public records. A matched control group selected from school health records was also studied. There was no difference between the two groups in the rate of school completion, contact with social authorities, or police contacts. The two groups did differ significantly, however, in the frequency of outpatient treatment. Thirty-one percent of the children with school phobia and 11% of the controls received outpatient treatment. Separation anxiety disorder and neurotic depression were commonly diagnosed in the school-phobic children.

Cantwell and Baker (1989) recently reported on a follow-up study of 151 children with a variety of DSM-III diagnoses (American Psychiatric Association 1980) who were initially referred to a community speech/language clinic. Thirty-one (20.5%) of these children were diagnosed with anxiety disorders: 9 had separation anxiety disorder, 14 had avoidant disorder, and 8 had overanxious disorder. These children received semiblind psychiatric evaluation 4 years later. Avoidant disorder was found to be the most stable of these childhood anxiety disorders. At follow-up, 4 (29%) of the children with avoidant disorder still had the same diagnosis, and another 4 (29%) with avoidant disorder were diagnosed as having overanxious disorder.

In contrast, four of the nine children with separation anxiety disorder were psychiatrically well at follow-up, and only one (11%) had a diagnosis of separation anxiety disorder at follow-up. This represents the highest rate of recovery among the anxiety disorders of childhood. Of all the children with anxiety disorders, the overanxious group ($n = 8$) had the lowest recovery rate, with only two children psychiatrically well at follow-up. However, the stability of overanxious disorder was also very low. Only two children had a persistent diagnosis of overanxious disorder, while another two had a follow-up diagnosis of avoidant disorder. According to this study, then, anxiety disorders among children are less stable and are associated with a higher rate of recovery than are the behavioral disorders.

Retrospective Studies

A number of researchers have focused on adults with anxiety disorder who also have a history of anxiety disorder during childhood. Berg et al. (1974) conducted a nationwide survey regarding childhood school phobia among 800 agoraphobic women in England and compared their findings with those obtained from 57 neurotic patients treated in an outpatient clinic. Both groups of patients reported a high frequency of school phobia (22%). The authors concluded that childhood school phobia is a precursor of later neurotic illness.

In a similar vein, Gittelman-Klein and Klein (1973) reported that 50% of adult agoraphobia and panic disorder patients retrospectively reported histories of fearfulness, dependency, separation anxiety, school adjustment difficulties, and phobias.

In another study, Klein et al. (1983) and Zitrin et al. (1983) interviewed patients who had been referred to an outpatient clinic for treatment of agoraphobia and simple phobia for a history of childhood separation anxiety. The female patients with agoraphobia reported separation anxiety more frequently both in childhood and adolescence than did patients with simple phobias (48% versus 15%, respectively). Curiously this relationship was absent among male agoraphobic patients. It is concluded from this study that agoraphobic women frequently suffered from separation anxiety disorder during childhood.

Natural History of Childhood Obsessive-Compulsive Disorder

This subject has been discussed in detail in Chapter 9. It has been consistently reported that adult obsessive-compulsive disorder often has its onset in childhood.

References

American Psychiatric Association: Diagnostic and Statistical Manual of Mental Disorders, 3rd Edition. Washington, DC, American Psychiatric Association, 1980

Berg I, Jackson A: Teenage school refusers grow up: a follow-up study of 168 subjects, ten years on average after in-patient treatment. Br J Psychiatry 47:366–370, 1985

Berg I, Butlar A, Richard J: Psychiatric illness in the mothers of school phobic adolescents. Br J Psychiatry 125:466–467, 1974

Berg I, Butlar A, Hall G: The outcome of adolescent school phobia. Br J Psychiatry 128:80–85, 1976

Cantwell DP, Baker L: Stability and natural history of DSM-III childhood diagnoses. J Am Acad Child Adolesc Psychiatry 28(5):691–700, 1989

Coolidge JC, Brodie RD, Feeney B: A ten-year follow-up study of sixty-six school phobic children. Am J Orthopsychiatry 34:675–684, 1964

Emde RN, Schmidt D: The stability of children's fears. Child Dev 49:1277–1279, 1978

Fischer M, Rolf JE, Hasazi JE, et al: Follow-up of a preschool epidemiological sample: cross-age continuities and predictions of later adjustment with internalizing and externalizing dimensions of behavior. Child Dev 55:137–150, 1984

Flakierska N, Lindstrom M, Gillberg C: School refusal: a 15–20 year follow-up study of 35 Swedish urban children. Br J Psychiatry 152:834–837, 1988

Gittelman-Klein R, Klein DF: School phobia: diagnostic considerations in the light of imipramine effects. J Nerv Ment Dis 156:199–215, 1973

Kagan J: Biological bases of childhood shyness. Science 240:167–171, 1988

Kagan J, Reznik JS, Snidman N: The physiology and psychology of behavioral inhibition in young children. Child Dev 58:1459–1473, 1987

Klein DF: Anxiety reconceptualized, in Anxiety: New Research and Changing Concepts. Edited by Klein DF, Rabkin J. New York, Raven, 1981, pp 235–262

Klein DF, Zitrin CM, Woerner MG, et al: Treatment of phobias, II: behavior therapy and supportive psychotherapy. Are there any supportive and specific ingredients? Arch Gen Psychiatry 40:139–145, 1983

Klein RG, Last CG: Anxiety Disorders in Children. Newbury Park, CA, Sage, 1989

MacFarlane JW, Allen L, Honzik MA: A Developmental Study of the Behavior Problems of Normal Children. Berkeley, CA, University of California Press, 1954

Miller LC, Barret CL, Hampe E: Comparison of reciprocal inhibition, psychotherapy, and waiting list control for phobic children. J Abnorm Psychol 79:269–279, 1972a

Morris DR, Sorokert E, Burruss G: Follow-up studies of shy withdrawn children. Evaluation of later adjustment. Am J Orthopsychiatry 24:743–754, 1954

Orvaschel H, Weissman MM: Epidemiology of anxiety disorders in children: a review, in Anxiety Disorders of Childhood. Edited by Gittelman R. New York, Guilford, 1986, pp 58–72

Reznik JS, Kagan J, Snidman N: Inhibited and uninhibited behavior: a follow-up study. Child Dev 51:660–680, 1986

Richman N, Stevenson J, Graham PJ: Preschool to School: A Behavioral Study. London, Academic, 1982

Roberts M: Persistent school refusal among children and adolescents. Life History Research in Psychopathology 4:79–198, 1975

Rodriguez A, Rodriguez M, Eisenberg L: The outcome of school phobia: a follow-up study based on 41 cases. Am J Psychiatry 116:540–544, 1959

Rosenbaum JF, Giederman J, Gersten M, et al: Behavioral inhibition in children of parents with panic disorder and agoraphobia. Arch Gen Psychiatry 45:463–470, 1988

Rutter M: Resilience in the face of adversity: protective factors and resistance to psychiatric disorder. Br J Psychiatry 147:598–611, 1985

Rutter M: Psychopathology and development: links between childhood and adult life, in Child and Adolescent Psychiatry: Modern Approaches, 2nd Edition. Edited by Rutter M, Herzov L. Oxford, Blackwell Scientific, 1986

Rutter M, Garmezy N: Developmental psychopathology, in Handbook of Child Psychiatry. Edited by Mussen PH. New York, John Wiley, 1983, pp 775–911

Rutter M, Tizard J, Whitmore K: Education, Health and Behaviour. New York, Krieger, 1981

Waldron S: The significance of childhood neurosis for adult mental health: a follow-up study. Am J Psychiatry 133:532–538, 1976

Weiss M, Burke A: A 5- to 10-year follow-up of hospitalized school phobic children and adolescents. Am J Orthopsychiatry 40:672–676, 1970

Zeitlen H: The natural history of psychiatric disorder in childhood. M.D. thesis, University of London, London, 1983

Zitrin CM, Klein DF, Woerner MG, et al: Treatment of phobias, I: comparison of imipramine hydrochloride and placebo. Arch Gen Psychiatry 40:125–138, 1983

Chapter 17

Theories of Etiology of Anxiety Disorders

A number of theoretical frames of reference are advanced in the literature to describe the etiology of anxiety disorders. In this chapter we will briefly discuss these theories.

Anxiety-like Disorders in Nonhuman Primates

Anxiety was once viewed as an exclusive characteristic of humans, who were seen as the only creatures with the cognitive and emotional abilities required to experience such a state (Kubie 1953). The current view (Suomi 1986) is that closely comparable analogues of anxiety (and anxiety disorders) exist in higher primates such as macaque or rhesus monkeys.

Most animal studies tend to correlate physiological signs with behavior patterns believed to denote anxiety. Increased activity of the adrenocortical system (Coe and Levine 1981; Levine 1983) and elevated heart rate and body temperature (Reite et al. 1981) have been linked with "anxious behavior."

The most relevant studies in monkeys tend to correlate maternal-infant separation with almost universal anxiety and fear on the part of the infant (Suomi et al. 1981). For the first several weeks or months, this anxiety appears to escalate, eventually either resolving or evolving to psychopathology. This research also suggests that a variety of experiences affects the monkeys' overall reaction to separation (either intensifying or reducing the severity of the experience), including the mother's disposition and the previous caregiver's interactions with the infant (e.g., neglectful or abusive versus caring and protective).

Age-related factors also are important, as adolescent monkeys respond much differently than do sibling infants to maternal separation (Mimeka et al. 1981). Essentially, these older monkeys react predictably and stereotypically with increased agitation and a relative decrease in vocalization (as opposed to infants, which will "coo" excessively once separated).

Some responses are also seen regardless of age group (Mendoza et al. 1978). For example, rhesus infants had significant increases in plasma cortisol output directly linked to activation of the hypothalamic-pituitary-adrenal axis. Scanlan (1984) also noted increased cortisol output under identical situations in both adolescent and adult monkeys, although the increase was not as marked. Various lines of evidence therefore suggest a common link in the physiological components of the anxiety reaction.

Certainly these and other studies give an indication that there is at least an analogous (if not homologous) relationship between humans and monkeys. Exploration of theoretical testing in primates is undoubtedly one step in the right direction toward a more complete understanding of anxiety and anxiety disorders.

Developmental Issues

Anxiety, per se, appears to exist as a normal adaptive mechanism aimed at increasing the conscious awareness of a dissonant situation, thus providing protection. It can, however, become maladaptive if it is excessive or improperly adjusted, thus inhibiting normal exploration and development.

It is well accepted (and documented) that behavioral concomitants of anxiety change with maturation. Because of the relatively inexact predictability of this change, behavior serves as a poor indicator of fear (Campbell 1986) and renders empirical investigation unreliable. This point must be considered in assessing the meaning and value of such research.

Ethological Theory of Development

This theory is based on the concept of a biologically based core response inherent in every behavior; the response is organized into adaptive systems aimed at maximizing the potential and survival of the species (Bowlby 1973; Charlesworth 1974). The suggestion is that genetic programming has maximum influence in the initiation of behavior, the influence of which is especially or even more crucial in the infant. For instance, crying and clinging are thought to ensure the proximity of the primary caregiver, thereby providing protection and nutrition (Ainsworth 1973). Along the same lines, behaviors such as clinging, smiling, and visual contact seem to initiate and prolong social sequences with adults (Stern 1974).

The development of fears is argued (Bowlby 1973) to be a mechanism designed for protection from predators and other harmful situations. At the root of this concept is the role of the primary attachment figure. If this person is responsive and available, then a sense of security develops. If this person is unavailable, increased anxiety and distress in the child are nearly always concomitant features. To go one step further, Bowlby (1973) hypothesized that fears in later life are residual from infantile fears that were based on a biological need for protection and nurturance.

Cognitive-Developmental Theory

Although certain fears (e.g., loud noises, quickly approaching or expanding objects) seem to elicit anxiety in the youngest infants, many fears require an association with a previous experience, usually one that is painful or results in some sort of separation (Lewis and Rosenblum 1974). Jones and Jones (1928) explained this as simple association or conditioning. It does seem apparent, however, that a certain degree of memory and anticipatory ability must exist to account for anxieties related to fears, e.g., of animals, strangers, or death.

This fear of the unknown, or of the strange, has generated much research activity and has been heralded by the nearly universal phenomenon of "stranger anxiety" in neonates (Spitz 1950). Authors have theorized that fear of novelty increases arousal (Berlyne 1960) and direct exploration and is directly involved in cognitive development (Flavell 1963). These ideas assume that once cognitive development begins (including object permanence and basic memory), infants become able to discriminate the familiar from the unfamiliar. Depending on his or her past experiences and environmental conditions, the infant will respond in a variety of different ways, ranging from casual wariness to a full-scale stress reaction.

Sroufe et al. (1974) advance this hypothesis one step further by suggesting that the recognition of discrepancy is only the first stage. They believe that contextual factors, as well as the infant's temperament and developmental level, will determine 1) whether the infant will respond, and if the infant does respond, 2) the manner of the response (i.e., positive or negative) and 3) the degree of response.

Despite the cogency of these explanations of fear, chronological and emotional development will consistently alter the objects of fear. Therefore, it is prudent to consider shifts in types and degrees of cognitive function when assessing fear and its development.

Learning Theories of Anxiety

Learning theories of behavior were originally adapted from Pavlov's (1927) conditioning model. In his model, Pavlov proposed that an early trauma initiates a mechanism (stimulus generalization) whereby one specific fear becomes the source of another.

Pavlov, however, was preceded by the experimenters Watson and Rayner (1920) in conducting the first published study on classical conditioning. "Albert B" was a small child conditioned to fear a previously neutral white rat by pairing its appearance with the clanging of a loud bell. Even after the bell's removal, Albert showed fear of the white rat that he had previously been unintimidated by. The researchers concluded that neurotic anxiety arises from events in which a neutral stimulus is serendipitously paired with an anxiety-provoking stimulus. This theory serves as the core principle for learning theorists. Serious objections to this theory have been raised, however, not the least of which is the inability to consistently duplicate the results. Because of this, new adaptations of this model have emerged.

Adaptive Evolutionary-Preparedness Theory

Initially proposed by Garcia and Koelling (1966) and later supported by Seligman (1970, 1971), the adaptive evolutionary-preparedness theory explains why relatively few stimuli induce phobia, as one might expect using only general learning theory. Essentially, the idea is that all *inherited* fears have specific object-relatedness that, when rated on a continuum of "preparedness," relates to a universal biological or survival value common to every individual. Preparedness is thus defined as that mechanism by which a more prepared fear is acquired more rapidly, is extinguished with greater difficulty and time, and is more resistant to explanation or rationalization. This model assumes that only the inherited value of certain fears enables them to produce intense anxiety.

Follow-up research has shown that "unprepared" stimuli are extinguished more rapidly than prepared stimuli. Clinical observations have shown this conclusion to be inaccurate, in that there are several reported cases of unprepared stimuli having created phobias that subsequently became extremely difficult to extinguish (Rachman and Seligman 1976). These apparent contradictions between theory and practice leave unexplained questions in the mind of the astute observer.

Psychodynamic Theories

Freudian concepts of anxiety are possibly the best known and least understood elements in the study of psychopathology. Freud (1893, 1894, 1917) postulated a trinomial system of classification. He believed that anxiety had at its roots 1) a response to danger, 2) separation from mother, and 3) anergic discharge. This last theory has all but been dropped from current ideologies (Compton 1972); we will therefore limit our discussion to the former two.

Anxiety as a Response to Danger

At first, Freud (1893) distinguished realistic anxiety (real "external" danger) from neurotic anxiety (internal danger, e.g., separation from a loved one). Later he dropped this explanation for the belief that helplessness is the essence of danger and that anxiety is the response of the ego to the threat of helplessness. He then cited five dangers that could precipitate an experience with helplessness: 1) birth, 2) loss of object, 3) loss of object's love, 4) loss of penis, and 5) loss of superego's love.

Anxiety then is viewed as a response to present or expected danger (internal or external), which then instigates physical and psychological defense processes. Most theorists would probably agree that the ego does not produce the anxiety as a signal of impending danger; rather, the ego recognizes and responds to danger while it modulates the impact of the anxiety.

Anxiety as a Response to Separation

Freud (1917) believed that separation (especially from mother) is first experienced at birth and that the effect of anxiety repeats the early impression of the act of birth. This does not imply that the infant is made anxious by birth, but that the birth experience itself is later reinstated in the effect of anxiety once the child acquires sufficient cognitive capacity to differentiate mother from strangers. Therefore, it is not until the eighth month or so, when an infant's cognitive abilities emerge, that the infant is able to experience separation anxiety.

Separation and stranger anxiety are distinct and independently occurring reactions (Bowlby 1969). Both require the cognitive ability to make differentiations, an attachment to a caregiver, and normal maturation (Emde et al. 1976). Freud went on to suggest that the ego comes to "tame" affect and to produce affect as a signal, serving as both an interpersonal and an intrapsychic communication modem. When an infant is faced with separation, then his or her screams not only signal a feeling of helplessness but also a preference for mother. Essentially Freud is saying that anxiety is best understood in terms of a communicative relationship between mother and self (object and self), whereby behavior is both promoted and inhibited.

Learning Theories

Another perspective is derived from learning theory. Shaffer (1986) depicts anxiety in instrumental terms as a secondary drive that is the conditioned part of fear. After acquisition of the emotional state from the pairing of fearful stimuli and subsequent successful escape, anxiety operates to mobilize the organism anew for avoidance of harm. What is learned can be subject to extinction. Thus, the behavioral therapy technique of deconditioning is understood within this conceptual framework.

Klein (1980) considers that psychoanalytic and learning theories are similar—recognizing, however, that both lack comprehensive explanations for the origin of anxiety. Recently, there has been an attempt to apply to anxiety the cognitive reconceptualization of depression. Beck and Emery (1985) have called attention to the possibility of a cognitive component of anxiety. They assert that an overemphasis on affect has characterized the early study of anxiety.

Unwittingly, this has obscured what may be the hallmark of anxiety: an underlying preoccupation with danger. As with the reconceptualization of depression, the thrust of this new perspective is a cognitive treatment approach to anxiety disorders.

Biological Theories

Biological theories of anxiety are also becoming more prevalent. Heightened interest in these theories developed from the observation that anxiety disorders tend to run in families. Twin studies demonstrated greater concordance for monozygotic than dizygotic twins for anxiety with panic attack but not for generalized anxiety (Torgersen 1983). Similar evidence has been found for the concordance of phobic disorders.

The long-standing debate surrounding centralist versus peripheralist theories of emotion has been enlightened by advances in state-of-the-art bioassay. Indeed, the debate has been overwhelmed or perhaps even superseded by the knowledge fostered by these technologies. The James-Lange theory (James 1884), paraphrased as "we run therefore we fear," maintained that it is the conscious awareness of the concomitants of arousal, such as rapid heart rate, that brings us to experience anxiety. Emotion, in this view, results from peripheral nervous system "cybernetics." The discovery of differential quantities of affect-related neurotransmitters in plasma in itself might seem empirical verification of the peripheral nervous system's role in the experience of emotion. Indeed, evidence is accumulating that persons with anxiety disorders are characterized by increased levels of circulating catecholamines. That is, anxious persons have higher concentrations of the agents that stimulate respiratory and cardiac activity—epinephrine and norepinephrine—in their blood.

Advances in our understanding of psychophysiology, however, challenge the ideas of central and peripheral nervous system orthogonality in emotion. What is now known about neurotransmitters—the systems' functional links—has obliged conceptual integration of the two systems.

Studies of the responses of anxious patients to provocative stimuli led investigators to examine the function of neurotransmitters in affective disorders. Research on the receptor sites of central neurotransmitters increased in importance. The beta-noradrenergic receptors have proven particularly significant in affective disorders. For example, depressed persons show supersensitivity of beta-*nor*adrenergic receptors (Carlson 1986). Beta-receptor sites are also implicated in anxiety disorders, and it is the *ad*renergic receptors that are linked to anxiety. In patients with anxiety disorder, the beta-adrenergic receptors are "downregulated" (Nesse et al. 1984). This suppression is thought to result from elevated levels of circulating catecholamines.

It is likely that the tacit historical influence of Walter Cannon brought investigators to seek central nervous system influences on the neurotransmitter/peripheral system dynamics in emotion. Cannon (1929) argued that emotions such as anxiety originate in the central nervous system. Thus, peripheral effects, such as increased respiration and cardiac output, are seen as epiphenomena.

The focus of contemporary research on the central nervous system origin of emotions is the locus coeruleus. Janowsky et al. (1982) found noradrenergic neurons at this site; they also implicated the locus coeruleus as the site of action of the commonly used antidepressants. Subsequent work linked this same area of the brain to adrenergic neurons and anxiety. It is now known that the same medication that influences the activity of the locus coeruleus will also block the occurrence of panic attacks among anxious patients.

There is also new understanding of the function of the neurotransmitter gamma-aminobutyric acid (GABA): it is linked to the effectiveness of the benzodiazepines in alleviating anxiety. GABA is a catalytic agent in the binding of a benzodiazepine to its receptor. The latter observation has generated a theoretical corollary: in terms of brain chemistry, the causal factor in anxiety disorder is an "impostor" substance that binds to receptors and that, under normal circumstances, is sensitive to benzodiazepines. Blocking of the benzodiazepine-dependent function at the receptor site results in a chemical milieu that induces the psychophysiological phenomenon of anxiety.

Correlational studies have linked mitral valve prolapse and panic disorder. Panic attacks, which induce autonomic stress, have been hypothesized to produce the structural mitral valve prolapse deformity. Alternatively, mitral valve prolapse and panic attacks may represent a basic generalized disturbance of autonomic function.

Clinical studies on the biological foundations for anxiety are new. Most research to date has involved adult participants, and analogues for children and adolescents are not yet in hand. Nevertheless, the phenomena cited are integral to physiological functioning. Refinements may be necessary, but age should not rule out such functional, causal relationships.

Physical Disability and Anxiety

Children with chronic physical illness are at higher risk for serious psychiatric impairment. If the brain is involved, the risk is even higher (Breslau 1985). Breslau showed the increased psychopathology in two categories: anxiety (regressive) and conflict with parents. Isolation was found to be more common in children with central nervous system involvement. Other studies (Mattar and Yaffe 1974; Wertheim 1978) have also reported emotional problems associated with chronic physical illness or disability, including anxiety, depression, low self-esteem, and increased emotional dependency.

References

Ainsworth MD: The development of infant mother attachment, in Review of Child Development Research, Vol 3. Edited by Caldwell B, Riccinte H. Chicago, IL, University of Chicago Press, 1973, pp 1–94

Beck AT, Emery G: Anxiety Disorders and Phobias: A Cognitive Perspective. New York, Basic Books, 1985

Berlyne DE: Conflict, Arousal and Curiosity. New York, McGraw-Hill, 1960

Bowlby J: Attachment (Attachment and Loss Series, Vol 1). New York, Basic Books, 1969

Bowlby J: Separation: Anxiety and Anger (Attachment and Loss Series, Vol 2). New York, Basic Books, 1973

Breslau N: Psychiatric disorders in children with physical disabilities. J Am Acad Child Psychiatry 24:87–94, 1985

Campbell SB: Developmental issues in childhood anxiety, in Anxiety Disorders of Childhood. Edited by Gittelman R. New York, Guilford, 1986, pp 24–57

Cannon WB: Bodily Changes in Pain, Hunger, Fear and Rage. New York, Appleton, 1929

Carlson NR: Physiology of Behavior, 3rd Edition. Boston, Allyn & Bacon, 1986

Charlesworth WR: General issues in the study of fear, in The Origins of Fear. Edited by Lewis M, Rosenbaum LA. New York, John Wiley, 1974, pp 249–268

Coe CL, Levine S: Normal responses to mother infant separation in non human primates, in Anxiety: New Research and Changing Concepts. Edited by Klein DF, Rabkin JG. New York, Raven, 1981

Compton AA: A study of psychoanalytic theory of anxiety, I: the development of Freud's theory of anxiety. J Am Psychoanal Assoc 20:3–44, 1972

Emde RN, Gaensbauer TJ, Harmon RJ: Emotional Expression in Infancy. New York, International Universities Press, 1976

Flavell J: The Developmental Psychology of Jean Piaget. Princeton, NJ, Van Nostrand Reinhold, 1963

Freud S: "Draft B" (1893), in The Standard Edition of the Complete Psychological Works of Sigmund Freud, Vol 1. Translated and edited by Strachey J. London, Hogarth Press, 1966, pp 179–184

Freud S: "Draft E." How anxiety originates (1894), in The Standard Edition of the Complete Psychological Works of Sigmund Freud, Vol 1. Translated and edited by Strachey J. London, Hogarth Press, 1966, pp 189–195

Freud S: Introductory lectures on psycho-analysis, lecture XXV: anxiety (1917), in The Standard Edition of the Complete Psychological Works of Sigmund Freud, Vols 15–16. Translated and edited by Strachey J. London, Hogarth Press, 1963, pp 392–411

Garcia J, Koelling RA: Relation of cue to consequences in avoidance learning. Psychonomic Science 4:123–124, 1966

James W: What is emotion? Mind 9:188–205, 1884

Janowsky A, Steranka LR, Gillespie D, et al: Role of neuronal signal input in the down regulation of central noradrenergic receptor function by antidepressant drugs. J Neurochem 39:290–292, 1982

Jones HE, Jones MC: Fear. Childhood Education 5:136–145, 1928

Klein DF: Anxiety reconceptualized, in Anxiety: New Research and Changing Concepts. Edited by Klein DF, Rabkin JG. New York, Raven, 1980, pp 235–262

Kubie LS: The concept of normality and neurosis, in Psychoanalysis and Social Work. Edited by Heinman M. New York, International Universities Press, 1953

Levine S: A psychobiological approach to the ontogeny of coping, in Stress Coping and Development in Children. Edited by Garmezy N, Rutter M. New York, McGraw-Hill, 1983, pp 107–131

Lewis M, Rosenblum LA (eds): The Origins of Fear. New York, John Wiley, 1974

Mattar ME, Yaffe SJ: Compliance of pediatric patients with therapeutic regimens. Postgrad Med 56(6):181–185, 1974

Mendoza SP, Smotherman WP, Miner M, et al: Pituitary adrenal response to separation in mother and infant squirrel monkeys. Dev Psychobiol 11:169–195, 1978

Mimeka S, Suomi SJ, Delizio RD: Multiple separations in adolescent monkeys: an opponent process interpretation. J Exp Psychol [Gen] 110:56–85, 1981

Nesse R, Cameron OG, Curtis GC, et al: Adrenergic function in patients with panic anxiety. Arch Gen Psychiatry 41:771–776, 1984

Pavlov I: Conditioned Reflexes. New York, Dover, 1927

Rachman S, Seligman MEP: Unprepared phobias: be prepared. Behav Res Ther 14:333–338, 1976

Reite M, Short R, Seiler C, et al: Attachment, loss and depression. J Child Psychol Psychiatry 22:141–169, 1981

Scanlan JM: Adrenocortical and behavioral responses to acute novel and stressful conditions: the influence of gonadal status, time course of response age and motor activity. Unpublished master's thesis, University of Wisconsin, Madison, 1984

Seligman M: On the generality of the laws of learning. Psychol Rev 77:406–418, 1970

Seligman M: Phobias and preparedness. Behav Ther 2:307–320, 1971

Shaffer D: Learning theories of anxieties, in Anxiety Disorders of Childhood. Edited by Gittelman R. New York, Guilford, 1986, pp 167–186

Spitz R: Anxiety in infancy: a study of its manifestation in the first year of life. Int J Psychoanal 31:537–544, 1950

Sroufe LA, Waters E, Matas L: Contextual determinants of infants' affective response, in The Origins of Fear. Edited by Lewis M, Rosenblum LA. New York, John Wiley, 1974, pp 49–72

Stern D: Mother and infant at play. The dyadic interaction involving facial, vocal and gaze behaviors, in The Effects of the Infant on Its Caregiver. Edited by Lewis M, Rosenblum LA. New York, John Wiley, 1974, pp 187–213

Suomi SJ: Anxiety-like disorders in young non-human primates, in Anxiety Disorders of Childhood. Edited by Gittelman R. New York, Guilford, 1986, pp 1–23

Suomi SJ, Kraemer GU, Baysinger M, et al: Inherited and experimental factors associated with individual differences in anxious behavior displayed by rhesus monkeys, in Anxiety: New Research and Changing Concepts. Edited by Klein DF, Rabkin JG. New York, Raven, 1981

Torgersen S: Genetic factors in anxiety disorders. Arch Gen Psychiatry 40:1085–1089, 1983

Watson J, Rayner R: Conditioned emotional reactions. J Exp Psychol 3:1–14, 1920

Wertheim ES: Developmental genesis of human vulnerability: conceptual re-evaluation, in The Child in His Family: Vulnerable Children, Vol 4. Edited by Anthony EJ, Koupernik C, Chiland C. New York, John Wiley, 1978, pp 17–36

Chapter 18

Conclusion

*T*he epidemiological studies of psychiatric disorders in children support the clinical observations that anxiety symptoms are commonly encountered in children and adolescents of both sexes (Kashani and Orvaschel 1990; Orvaschel and Weissman 1986). However, the empirical studies of anxiety disorders in children focusing on etiology, phenomenology, epidemiology, and treatment efficacies are scant and do not provide conclusive evidence to permit the attainment of the ultimate goal of providing specific treatment interventions. The advances made thus far, however, are noteworthy and promising.

The first formal effort to systematize the various categories of childhood anxiety disorders and specific diagnostic criteria for each category was presented in DSM-III (American Psychiatric Association 1980). This development stimulated a number of studies that generated data addressing the issue of reliability of the overall diagnostic category of childhood anxiety disorders (Mezzich and Mezzich 1985; Williams and Spitzer 1980; J.S. Werry, R.J. Methren, J. Fitzpatrick, unpublished observations, 1984). Although these studies obtained markedly different levels of agreement for the general category of childhood anxiety disorders and reported poor reliability, each of these studies was handicapped by a small sample size, which can seriously inflate or deflate coefficients of agreement (Last 1988).

Two studies that used larger samples did in fact reveal good to excellent reliability for the diagnostic category of childhood anxiety disorders (Last et al. 1987; J.S. Werry, R.J. Methren, J. Fitzpatrick, unpublished observations, 1984). Several clinical studies and case reports have provided data to support the "face" validity of the subcategories of childhood anxiety disorder such as separation anxiety disorder and overanxious disorder. It is felt that the distinction between separation anxiety and overanxious disorder may not be clear, and more data are needed on validity of these diagnoses.

The link between childhood anxiety disorders and adult anxiety disorders has interested researchers for some time. For example, convincing data suggest that the children of patients with agoraphobia or panic disorder often manifest separation anxiety (Weissman et al. 1984). Retrospective observations have also been made about the onset of adult anxiety disorder in childhood (e.g., Tyrer and Tyrer 1974). What are lacking, however, are longitudinal studies of children or adolescents with anxiety disorders that are pertinent to understanding the degree to which childhood disorders are precursors of adult anxiety disorders. The data on linkage between childhood obsessive-compulsive disorder and adult obsessive-compulsive disorder are more convincing and consistent.

The unstructured interview is still the most popular method for assessing anxiety in children. It has the advantage of comprehensiveness and flexibility but suffers from lack of reliability and validity (Werry 1986). Behavioral assessment methods, in contrast, are reliable yet contain inherent constraints. It may be more profitable to obtain direct evidence on internal data rather than inferring it from behaviors. Current self-report measures tend to be more specific than general and are often derived from adult forms (Peterson et al. 1988). It is important to note that use of self-report instruments with children assumes that the child is competent linguistically and cognitively and is willing to respond to the best of his or her ability. Other available instruments for the assessment of anxiety include structured interviews and physiological measures. Unfortunately, there is low reliability among the various measures (Werry 1986).

Proponents of developmentally based diagnostic frameworks clearly agree that there are continuities in some types of psychopathology during childhood. For example, Sroufe et al. (1983) found that avoidance of the caregiver as infants predicted preschoolers' later excessive dependency on the teacher. Literature and research data on children's fears and anxieties in nonclinical samples (Campbell 1986) are also very scant.

A number of researchers have advanced a number of theoretical constructs to explain the etiology of anxiety disorders. Most of these theories are based on the studies conducted in adults, but the data are applicable to children. It is felt on the basis of the current data that a variety of factors, alone or in combination, may underlie anxiety disorders in children. Stressful life events, heredity, and familial environmental factors all are said to play a role. Future investigation will clarify these roles and provide information on how specific stressors may produce specific categories of anxiety disorder: for example, separation from an attachment figure in early life may produce separation anxiety disorder in children.

It is still questionable as to how insecurity and anxiety manifest themselves at different ages and whether or not timid and anxious preschoolers develop into socially withdrawn fourth graders (Campbell 1986). Thus, longitudinal studies addressing these issues are needed.

A number of treatment modalities have been used over the span of this century, and each has produced inconsistent results. The current focus on psychopharmacotherapy is based on the success of drug treatment in adults who have panic disorder with agoraphobia. In children, only limited supportive evidence is available for the efficacy of this drug treatment. Clomipramine for the treatment of obsessive-compulsive disorder has been found to be consistently effective. The early claims for effectiveness of imipramine in the treatment of separation anxiety disorder are now being questioned by some researchers. Alprazolam therapy has been tried only rarely in children and has produced good results, without the withdrawal symptoms observed in adults.

In summary, the childhood anxiety disorders are a valid, exciting, and almost unfathomed field of inquiry waiting for researchers young and old to unravel their psychobiological web.

References

American Psychiatric Association: Diagnostic and Statistical Manual of Mental Disorders, 3rd Edition. Washington, DC, American Psychiatric Association, 1980

Campbell S: Developmental issues in childhood anxiety, in Anxiety Disorders of Childhood. Edited by Gittelman R. New York, Guilford, 1986, pp 24–57

Kashani JH, Orvaschel H: A community study of anxiety in children and adolescents. Am J Psychiatry 147:313–318, 1990

Last CG: Anxiety disorders in childhood and adolescence, in Handbook of Anxiety Disorders. Edited by Last CG, Hersen M. New York, Pergamon, 1988, pp 531–540

Last CG, Hersen M, Kazdin AE, et al: Psychiatric illness in the mothers of anxious children. Am J Psychiatry 144:1580–1583, 1987

Mezzich AC, Mezzich JE: Reliability of DSM-III vs DSM-II in child psychopathology. J Am Acad Child Psychiatry 24:273–280, 1985

Orvaschel H, Weissman MM: Epidemiology of anxiety disorders in children: a review, in Anxiety Disorders of Childhood. Edited by Gittelman R. New York, Guilford, 1986, pp 58–72

Peterson L, Burbach DJ, Chaney J: Developmental issues, in Handbook of Child Psychiatric Diagnosis. Edited by Last CG, Hersen M. New York, John Wiley, 1988, pp 463–482

Sroufe LA, Fox N, Pancake V: Attachment and dependency in developmental perspective. Child Dev 54:1615–1627, 1983

Tyrer P, Tyrer S: School refusal, truancy, and adult neurotic illness. Psychol Med 4:416–421, 1974

Weissman MM, Leckman JR, Merikangar KR, et al: Depression and anxiety disorders in parents and children: results from the Yale Family Study. Arch Gen Psychiatry 41:845–852, 1984

Werry JS: Diagnosis and assessment, in Anxiety Disorders of Childhood. Edited by Gittelman R. New York, Guilford, 1986, pp 73–100

Williams JBW, Spitzer RL: DSM-III field trials: interrater reliability and list of project staff and participants (Appendix F), in Diagnostic and Statistical Manual of Mental Disorders, 3rd Edition. Washington, DC, American Psychiatric Association, 1980, pp 467–481

Index